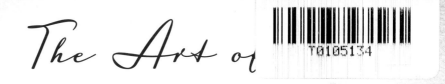

The Art of

AYURVEDIC NUTRITION

Ancient Wisdom for Health, Balance, and Dietary Freedom

Susie Colles, PhD

Skyhorse Publishing

Skyhorse Publishing books may be purchased in bulk at special discounts for sales promotion, corporate gifts, fund-raising, or educational purposes. Special editions can also be created to specifications. For details, contact the Special Sales Department, Skyhorse Publishing, 307 West 36th Street, 11th Floor, New York, NY 10018 or info@skyhorsepublishing.com.

Skyhorse® and Skyhorse Publishing® are registered trademarks of Skyhorse Publishing, Inc.®, a Delaware corporation.

Visit our website at www.skyhorsepublishing.com.

10 9 8 7 6 5 4 3 2 1

Library of Congress Cataloging-in-Publication Data is available on file.

Cover design by Daniel Brount
Cover illustrations by Iku Baishya

Print ISBN: 978-1-5107-4902-3
Ebook ISBN: 978-1-5107-4903-0

Printed in China

For Ma

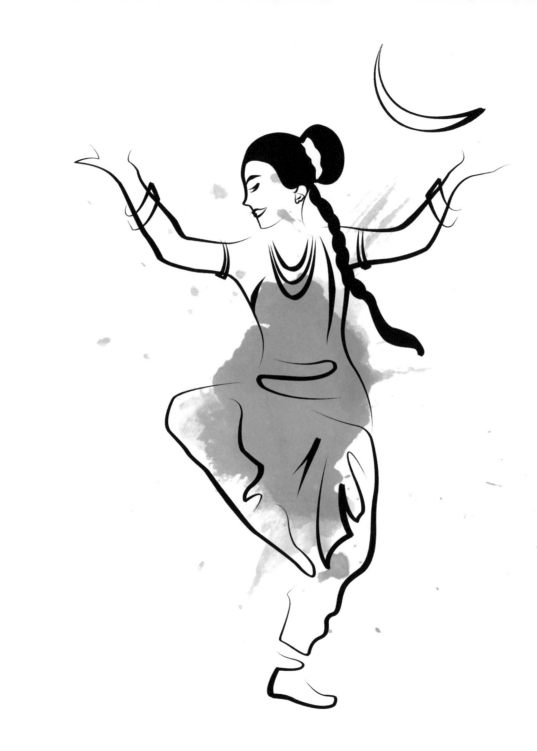

Table of Contents

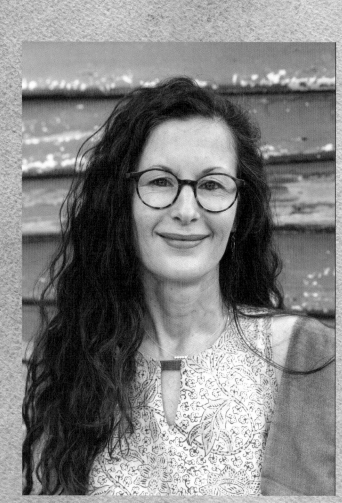
©Lisa Colles Photography

About the Author

Susie Colles is a dietitian turned natural health practitioner on a journey. During her thirty-year career she completed a Bachelor of Science in human movement; a Master's degree in nutrition and dietetics; a PhD that examined links between weight management, eating behavior, metabolism, and psychology; more than twelve hundred hours of formal *Āyurveda* study under experienced Indian and Western Ayurvedic doctors; and published a dozen peer-reviewed scientific papers. She has worked as a fitness expert; a clinical dietitian specializing in diabetes, kidney disease, gastrointestinal disorders, cystic fibrosis, and aged care; a weight loss counselor working with people one-on-one and in groups; a health researcher; university lecturer; public speaker; health writer; international volunteer in women's health; yoga therapist, and Ayurvedic practitioner. At the personal level, Susie has lived the diet mentality, and suffered debilitating sinus pain, inflammatory bowel disease, and migraines—all partly aggravated and healed by diet. Experiencing people's struggles and frustrations, she has reflected deeply on what, how, and why people eat; what causes disease; and ever-broadening definitions of health.

Having trained and worked in the West, it was only after moving to India and formally studying *Āyurveda*, that the science and art of nutritional healing truly resonated for Susie. Personally, she found therapeutic answers, established a profound relationship with food, a naturally comfortable body weight, and ever-deepening sense of health. Today she works as a yoga therapist and Ayurvedic health practitioner, with entire beings, within social settings and natural cycles, offering ideas and practices to guide balanced health, self-knowledge, and spiritual freedom. Susie grew up in Australia; has lived in Europe, Africa, and Asia; and currently lives in the hills of Southern India. Find her website at susiecolles.com.

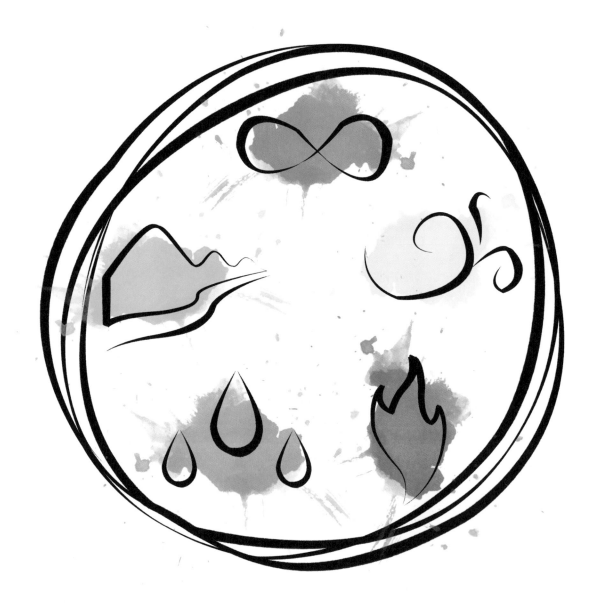

Introduction

This book guides the art of Ayurvedic food-related wisdom through the application of theory and practice, aiming to balance the physical body and in turn support the mind and emotions, the flow of vital energy, intuitive intelligence, and spirit. The ancient Indian system of *Āyurveda* is a natural, holistic healing system that is highly relevant to the mounting food-health challenges of today. The Ayurvedic approach to lifelong health centers around the *dosha*—three intelligent bodily managers that mix within us to determine our unique metabolic constitution. Understanding our personal constitution offers deep insights into our nature, and is key to making dietary and lifestyle choices that support physical balance and mental happiness.

The body is a miraculous, intelligent vessel—quite out of common awareness its base functions are self-maintaining. The physical body grounds us and acts as our base and touchstone to tangible, sensual existence. When its functions are balanced, the body fills with vitality and joy. If we listen, the body is a constant teacher, yet subtle voices telling us how the body feels are seldom truly noted. We often hold little faith in the physical body, and don't offer it the attention or support it deserves. When the machinery does its job, the body is a workhorse that toils toward the mind's aspirations. We expect the same performance, day in, day out, regardless of physical limits and natural cycles. Sometimes the body feels like a burden. Feeding it, cleaning it, and putting up with its pains, noises, and smells can make us forget its living, illuminated intelligence. When balanced, the physical body is completely geared toward life. A doctor or healer may offer a boost, but it's the nature of the body to heal. Health and happiness come from within.

Our body may seem familiar to us, but the body changes so rapidly that constancy is just an illusion. Every morning we look in the mirror at a different entity. Moment by moment, the physical body performs thousands, possibly millions of simultaneous functions, synthesizing and metabolizing compounds precisely as the need arises. Skin and gut tissues slough off and are regenerated. Millions of cells die and birth simultaneously. The body's main constituent, water, flows continuously through all living tissues. The foods we ate yesterday are becoming bodily tissues today. Metabolic wastes build up and are removed. The ability of the physical body to continually adapt to changing conditions is one of its most elegant features.

Modern medicine tries to understand the physical body through orchestrated scientific trials, based on the fact that humans are a series of interwoven biological compounds undergoing elegantly transforming reactions, powered by calories, predetermined by genes. This way of knowing the human body divides it into ever-smaller parts, and hands the power of knowledge to science and medicine. *Āyurveda* understands the physical body as one aspect of a greater whole. As a material entity, the physical body is comprised fundamentally of the five great states of matter: earth, water, fire, air, and ether. These five elements that comprise the human body also comprise all planetary matter and can

be experienced and understood by everyone. How does the body accumulate these elements? Through the foods we eat. In Sanskrit, the ancient language of India that directly connects sounds with forms, the term for body, *sharira*, refers to the entity needing constant replenishment. All physical tissues need constant feeding, waste removal, cleansing, maintenance, replacement, and rejuvenation from wear and tear.

More than the physical body we see and identify with, the ancient traditions of *Āyurveda*, yoga, and Chinese medicine also understand the body as a system of energy flowing through subtle channels that obey universal laws. Traditional Chinese medicine knows this flowing energy as *qi*. In *Āyurveda*, and its sister science, yoga, the body's vital energy is known as *prāna*, the intelligent force that enlivens every aspect of our system and all life on Earth. *Prāna* is not personal. It's a common pasture to which all beings have equal rights. *Prāna* can be awakened and enhanced within us as individuals; and universally it's a common pasture to which all beings have equal rights. In modern life, the primary ways we take in fresh *prāna* are through our thoughts, feelings, and actions; our social and wider environment; and breath (air), the sun, water, and food. The elements that comprise the physical body, and the energy that vitalizes it, can't be artificially separated within us or from the external environment.

More specifically, *Āyurveda* and yoga see each human lives within five energy envelopes or sheaths. Each sheath supports a different aspect of life. The innermost sheath is the physical body, made up mainly of the two heaviest elements, earth and water. The physical body is constructed from the foods we eat, the fluids we drink, and the air we breathe, and is referred to as the *food body*. The food body is the densest and most slowly vibrating sheath. Within and around the food body exist four progressively more subtle, vibrating fields.

Next, and lighter in density, is the *vital body*, also known as the breath or *prānic* sheath. It is through the vital body that the life-force *prāna* flows—through channels known as *nādis* (meridians in Chinese medicine), and also through the *chakra* system, energetic wheels or transformers that store and release flowing energy. Yogic texts speak of 72,000 subtle channels, and 114 chakras within the human energy network. The development, organization, and vibrancy of the physical and mental bodies particularly depends on the *prānic* sheath.

More subtle in density is the *mental body* or envelope, the channel through which the mind's thoughts and emotions move. Western medicine tends to think of the mind as the brain, whereas *Āyurveda* sees the mind as a subtle sheath, permeating and moving throughout the entire physical body. Plus, the mind extends outside the physical body, to wherever we consciously focus. Our dietary patterns directly affect the food body, vital body, and the mental sheath.

Enveloping these three bodies is the even-more-refined *wisdom body*, or sheath of intuitive knowledge. This vibrating field relates to the subconscious and unconscious mind, and connects us to multidimensional knowing, including intuition and higher awareness. And the final and most subtle body is known as the *bliss body*, or transcendental sheath. The bliss body envelops the wisdom, mental, vital, and food bodies. It is the field of the soul or spirit, our innermost and outermost universal connection. The bliss body is the aspect of being that resonates with pure consciousness.

The five bodies

When all five bodies exist in harmony, health flourishes. In their arrangement, each body supports the other and contributes to all aspects of the whole being. All bodies influence our physical being, and the food body influences every other aspect. Life is a combination of the physical body, mind and senses, vital force, wisdom, and reincarnating soul. Health encompasses all of these aspects.

Translated from its Sanskrit origin, the root *ayus* represents the intelligent combination of the body, sense organs, mind, and soul that together provide life and continuity of consciousness. In *Āyurveda* the term *ayur* denotes this life as dynamic, creative, and multidimensional; a principle spanning constant evolution and change. From the root *vid*, meaning knowledge or to know, the word *veda* relates to a rational progression of knowledge, often translated as "science," but *veda* refers to knowledge derived coherently from experience rather than the logic-based "facts" lauded by modern science. A living wisdom that offers understanding through direct observation and conscious involvement. Birthed in India, for many millennia—and arguably more relevant today— *Āyurveda* offers a complete natural science of life, virtuous living, and healthy longevity.

When constantly fatigued or "under the weather," we may seek health, but don't know how to find it, or even how to describe it. In Western systems, medical professionals are trained to see clinical conditions and diseases, defined by the presence of measurable symptoms; and *health* becomes the absence of clinically measurable disease. Subtle facets of the body, our daily routine and living environment, and whether we actually *feel* healthy, are not things modern tests examine. In contrast, *Āyurveda* doesn't focus on specific disease states and symptomatic treatments. *Āyurveda* is a life-positive approach, with *health* as the emphasis—a thriving, wholly conscious, and connected way of being, achieved through balancing one's unique constitution with complementary foods and daily routines, living in harmony with Mother Nature, and through simplicity, happiness, and elevation of spirit.

This book consists of two parts. Part I focuses more on theory and introduces key Ayurvedic principles. Part II concentrates on putting these theories and principles into practice. Part I, Chapter 1 journeys into the background and evolution of *Āyurveda*, and describes how Mother Nature, who in *Āyurveda* is the principle of material nature, supports human development and health. Chapter 1 appreciates Mother Nature's five great elements that comprise this planet and our physical self. We examine the qualities of each of these elements, and begin to understand them in ourselves. We also consider Mother Nature's cycles, and how cosmic cycles govern our physical well-being.

In Chapter 2, the focus moves to the body's three subtle managers, or *dosha*—*vāta*, *pitta*, and *kapha*. We get to know the *dosha* and launch an expedition into our own unique constitution. The health model of the three *dosha* is a concept that is central and unique to *Āyurveda*. The *dosha* are three intelligent, complimentary forces that guide all physical function and form. Subtle in nature, we can't always see them, but we can see the results of their actions. In each body, all three *dosha* exist in various intensities and proportions. By understanding our unique combination of *dosha*, our physical and mental tendencies become clearer, and we gain a personal ongoing methodology for balancing health. When our personal mix of the three *dosha* function harmoniously, the physical body operates seamlessly, and upholds all aspects of life. But if the *dosha* become vitiated and lose equilibrium, the physical body loses integrity, and imbalance and disease descend. For *Āyurveda*, imbalance within these three subtle managers is the root cause of disease. What can imbalance the *dosha*? Just about anything! Everything internal and external is a potential source of health, and also a potential source for disease—it depends on the

dose and qualities of the would-be substance or action, and the daily, seasonal, and constitutional needs of the individual. In general, three main precipitators of *dosha* imbalance exist. One factor is the impact of time. Time's effects include the aging process and changing seasons. We work against time by denying the process of aging; by being out of sync with natural cycles— when we eat unseasonal foods or warming foods in summer heat, when we eat too often or irregularly, or eat at a time when the digestive fires are weak. Our timing is off when we make choices based on past conditioning rather than present conditions. Another disease precipitator is the mind. Logic and reason offer incredible possibilities, but the intellect is limited. According to *Āyurveda*, many poor dietary and lifestyle choices, and *dosha* and digestive imbalance occur due to *prājñāparādha*, a Sanskrit term that translates to "mistake of intellect" or even "crimes against wisdom." We enter its grip when we knowingly or unwittingly choose foods or actions that don't suit us. We choose heavy foods when the body asks for light, eat more than is comfortable, or in the absence of bodily hunger. The mind aggravates the *doshas* and initiates disease when we think untoward and excessive thoughts, generate or suppress strong emotions, will the body beyond its capacity, ignore or forcibly stimulate natural urges, and through our ignorance and delusions. The sense impressions we take in through the eyes, ears, nose, tongue, and skin are a third significant cause of *dosha* imbalance. The senses are our windows to the world, but they are often abused or distracted. Underuse, overuse, or misuse occurs when we eat food dominated by one or two tastes or textures; consume physically and chemically manipulated foods; and excessively expose ourselves to lights, sounds, or synthetic or tight clothing. Sight is the dominant sense, but the eyes are easily fooled. And the tongue, nose, and skin are enfeebled. According to *Āyurveda*, anything taken into the system that is incompletely processed is carried within us and becomes a potential seed of disease. When the senses are not in order and discernment is not strong, incomplete impressions foster imbalance. Many of us stockpile sensory experiences and grievances that never fully heal.

The potential initiators of illness are many. The scriptures tell us most diseases—eighty categories—are *vāta* in origin, next comes *pitta dosha* with forty categories, and then *kapha*, which initiates twenty types of disease. As imbalance takes hold, *Āyurveda* sees the disease process occur in six stages toward full-blown manifestation. In the first and second stages of the disease process, one *dosha* becomes aggravated and begins to accumulate and rise in its home-site—*kapha's*

primary home site is the stomach, *pitta* lives in the small intestine, and *vāta* resides in the colon. As a *dosha* becomes aggravated, the body's natural intelligence produces an aversion to factors that will increase the *dosha* further, and an attraction to substances and actions with opposite, pacifying qualities. When feeling hot and dry, we get out of the sun, and seek out a cool glass of water. On a cold gusty night, we close the windows and crave a hearty, warming meal. The body seeks stability and balance. Correcting early *dosha* imbalance prevents illness before it flourishes. But when minor problems go unaddressed and the body's wisdom is not respected, conditions deepen and spread. In the third and fourth stages of the disease process, the aggravated *dosha* spreads out of the gut and adjacent areas into the circulation, eventually finding a weak tissue or organ, or system that shares an affinity to settle in, multiply, and deposit toxins and wastes. Around this time, we often become aware of uncomfortable symptoms and Western medicine looks in—symptom-by-symptom, organ-by-organ, drug-by-drug—although the problem started upstream. Ayurvedic wisdom recognizes physical symptoms—the aches, inflammations, unruly blood tests, weight gain, tissue growth, and organ disorders—as observable consequences of causes originating somewhere else. It is during the third and fourth stages that the body's natural intelligence becomes silenced, and self-balance is no longer sought. Even though the body needs rebalancing, we are no longer compelled toward it. Although certain substances and actions harm us, we no longer move away. Instead, ironically, regrettably, we crave the things that make us ill. The body is accustomed to them, and they regale the senses and provide a short-term lift. Wayward intelligence does much to explain our fondness for highly processed, devitalized foods, and why many ailments endure. In the fifth and sixth stages of the disease process, disorders intensify, spread, and become difficult to cure. Chronic conditions set in.

To intercept the trajectory of chronic disease, one art of Ayurvedic nutrition is choosing foods to balance each unique *dosha* mix, detailed in Chapter 3. *Āyurveda* reads bodies and matches foods; choosing food to complement each body, beginning with six dominant tastes: sweet, sour, salty, pungent, bitter, and astringent. Certain tastes balance certain *dosha* and are encouraged, but health prospers when all six tastes are eaten daily. Among other qualities, foods heat and cool the body, bring moisture or dryness, and attributes of heavy and light. We explore these ideas, plus three other universal qualities present in the foods we eat—*sattva, rajas,* and *tamas*—that primarily affect the mind. Of these,

sattva is an innate balancing and harmonizing force that lives in us all, yet is easily obscured. The remainder of Chapter 3 explores the main food group and many specific foods, considering their dominant qualities and potential to influence the *dosha*. We examine the benefits of different eating patterns to enhance *dosha* balance, and nutritional and holistic health.

Thousands of years ago, when *Āyurveda* was born, the food supply—and world—were different, but even then, *Āyurveda* knew that food plays a fundamental role in health. Western science is just beginning to appreciate the potential of diet to provoke disease or support health, and recently discovered the significance of the gut microbiome—legions of bacteria and fungi that inhabit the gut, enabling digestion, immunity, and robust mental well-being. The central function of food and the gut has been long understood by *Āyurveda*. The *Taittirīya Upanishad*, an ancient Vedic text, states "All that exists on earth is born of *anna* (food), lives on *anna*, and in the end merges into *anna. Anna* indeed is the first born amongst all beings. Therefore it is called the universal medicine."[1] Food enables and holds life together. *Annam Brahma*—food is god.

The ability to digest the foods we eat is another central theme of *Āyurveda*. Chapter 4 inspects, befriends, and stokes the *agni*, or digestive fires. Agriculture makes mud and manure into food. Digestion makes food into energy and tissues. What is on our plate one day, is bodily tissue the next. We live in active partnership with the compounds we consume. From food, through the grace of the digestive *agni*, *Āyurveda* sees that seven distinct tissues are created in a particular order. First plasma, then blood, muscle, fat, bone, marrow, and finally reproductive tissues. When the digestive fires are strong, all tissues are nourished, the reproductive cells are well-formed, and *ojas* arises. *Ojas* is the most refined and nutritive essence of food; life force in a liquid medium. This subtle nectar is fed back to the body, enhancing all functions, underpinning immunity, resilience, and health.

Too little food, too much food, or foods the gut can't handle, disturbs the digestion and metabolism, and promotes the buildup of undigested toxins, or *āma*. As well as examine digestion, Chapter 4 appreciates the probable presence of undigested toxins in life. To *Āyurveda*, poor dietary habits, weak digestion, and the presence of undigested toxins play a central role in disease. Two generations ago, illnesses such as diabetes, cancer, attention deficit disorder, arthritic conditions, and thyroid dysfunction affected an unfortunate few. Never before have humans suffered concurrently from malnutrition and obesity—both conditions present at the same time, in the same individual. Today, many adults and children lack robust immunity, and fewer people age gracefully, enjoying a functional, full life. Food builds the food body, and the foods we eat, and the ways we eat them, contribute to either health or disease.

From an Ayurvedic perspective, poor dietary choices and poor digestion are common causes of imbalances and toxins that make us more susceptible to chronic inflammation; high blood pressure; disturbed blood fats; insulin resistance; diabetes; weight gain; immune dysfunction; autoimmune disease; menstrual disorders; conditions of the heart and circulatory system, lungs and respiratory system, liver and digestive system, kidneys and urinary system, ovaries and reproductive system, hormonal and nervous systems; many cancers; and degenerative and chronic health conditions—all especially relevant today. At every level, we are what we do, and do not, digest.

To support the healing of modern-day problems of weight gain and debility, Chapter 5 offers insights into *langhana* and *brimhana*, the reducing and building natures of certain foods that work to reduce and lighten, or build and strengthen, the food body. In life, all possibilities—from comfortable mobility, to a good night's sleep, to mental clarity, attainment of our highest potential, true contentment, and longevity—are contingent on health, and are also markers of it. Weight gain is not an issue of too many calories; a thyroid problem is not just an issue of the gland. Good health and good nutrition encompass the whole body, and also lie beyond its borders. Seeking health through stand-alone nutrients or the treatment of sovereign parts, fragments and distances us from life at large.

How we relate to food and the food environment influences what, why, how, and when we eat, and our ability to derive goodness and vitality from food. In Chapter 6 we examine embodied eating, a universally relevant concept to help us more clearly and wholly perceive the foods we eat and how they affect the body. Embodied eaters bring the mind and senses into the body to look, listen, and feel more deeply in order to know what's truly going on; and in deepening their food relations, nurture greater respect and gratitude for our near and far connections with food.

Part II focuses on practice. Chapter 7 teaches how to embrace Mother Nature's daily and seasonal cycles. The mind has been taught guidelines: eat this; don't eat that. But the body knows none of these rules. While constant flux is natural, *routines* and *cycles* support physical health; living according to universal rhythms and laws. Along these lines, Chapter 7 also looks at the universal importance and practice of eating foods that are seasonal, local, and fresh.

In Ayurvedic health and healing, maintaining or restoring the strength of digestion is key. Chapter 8 pays further homage to the digestive fires, advises how to stoke them, and examines methods to remove undigested toxins, or *āma*. These two steps are fundamental and often primary in moving toward *dosha* balance.

Chapter 9 returns to the *dosha*, providing detailed guidance on living for balance, including finer points on balancing tastes, foods, qualities, and eating patterns. Examples of meal plans and lifestyle choices are given for each of the three *dosha*. And we return to the quality of *sattva*, a balancing, harmonizing force that when nurtured, enhances the intelligence and metabolism of all constitutions. Guidance is provided on eating and living *sattva*.

In Chapter 10 we delve into the practice of embodied eating, and learn to look more wholly and deeply. Following the wisdom of Mother Nature, the wisdom and messages of the whole body, and wisdom consolidated through personal experience are significant themes of *Āyurveda*. Rather than taking eating and health cues from outside ourselves, moving toward physical balance entails looking, listening, feeling, practicing, and experiencing for ourselves. Throughout Chapter 10, you will learn to use personal observations to cultivate self-knowledge and self-awareness, and inform relevant choices. Outmoded attitudes and habits are anti-transformation, but with awareness, each decision becomes an opportunity for growth and change. With fresh eyes, we examine and conquer the secret life of hunger, and decode food cravings. We inspect the food body's waste products, interpret the language of the tongue, awaken and manage the senses and mind, and invite the light of intuition. Rather than depend solely on logic, we incorporate *feeling* into daily food choices, and truly live each experience. Chapter 10 concludes with conscious cookery, getting to know food and elevate the eating experience, plus consideration of our food relations, and how to offer food the gratitude and reverence it deserves.

To consolidate change, in Chapter 11 we delve into habituation, or *satmya*, and the secret life of habits. Old patterns are looked in the eye and then let go, in order to focus on new habits that support and balance the *dosha*. We also appreciate the significance of fostering congruous connections through social and environmental supports. To complement this nutritional guide, a final appendix offers cooking tips and recipes, followed by a bibliography and references.

For Westerners steeped in biomedical science and nutrition, *Āyurveda* provides new organizing principles to describe and understand our own bodies and the world around us. It offers a framework that preserves the integrated nature of the universe, while supporting each individual to navigate their own path. Habits of thought and action are highly personal; a personal culture, if you will. *The Art of Ayurvedic Nutrition* invites you to expand your personal and food culture, and in doing so expand your ethos of the physical body, health, disease, healing, your surroundings, and even your innermost nature. Grounded in wisdom, theory, and practice, this book empowers you with principles of the living intelligence of *Āyurveda*. Working toward holistic balance (rather than single pieces of the puzzle), encourages displaced fragments to move gently, spontaneously back to natural, harmonious living. Sound good? Let's get started!

PART I

Ayurvedic Principles

The first half of this book examines key Ayurvedic principles that underpin the theory of eating for healthy balance.

Āyurveda was birthed in India yet its truest origins are speculative and difficult to reference in time. At present, the wisdom and practice of *Āyurveda* is represented in three main scriptures. The earliest comprehensive work dealing purely with *Āyurveda* is the *Charaka Samhitā*, conceived in seven encyclopedic volumes well over two thousand years ago. The *Charaka Samhitā* focuses on the immediate and distant causes of disease, the signs of disease and health, and therapeutic treatments. The second significant text, the *Sushruta Samhitā*, believed to have been recorded a few hundred years after the *Charaka Samhitā*, focuses on

surgical treatments and general medicine. And in more recent times, around twelve hundred years ago, sage writer *Vāgbhata* analyzed, condensed, and presented the teachings of these two scriptures in a third major treatise known as the *Ashtanga Hridayam*, meaning heart of the eight branches of *Āyurveda*. These three texts, the *Charaka Samhitā*, *Sushruta Samhitā*, and *Ashtanga Hridayam* form the major triad of knowledge of Ayurvedic medicine. In more recent centuries, numerous *nighantus* or accessory texts have been added on subjects including pathology, diagnosis, new medicinal herbs, and foods. And in recent decades, a number of Indian and Western doctors, practitioners, and commentators have contributed to these teachings through their learning and experience. I have drawn on all these sources in formulating the key Ayurvedic principles communicated in this book, and also my own education and practice, with particular deference to the wisdom of the *Charaka Samhitā*. Further details of guiding references appear in the bibliography at back.

The first written record of *Āyurveda* appears among the ancient Vedic scriptures. The oldest of these texts, the *Rig Veda* (Sanskrit for "in praise of knowledge") dates back over four thousand five hundred years, where within one hundred twenty-eight hymns devoted to spiritual attainment, the five great elements and many herbs and medical practices are described. The youngest of the four *Vedas*, the *Atharva Veda,* recorded over three thousand two hundred years ago, promotes a disease-free life and longevity through spiritual observances and rites, and also records the earliest known ideas on human anatomy, along with descriptions of diseases and medical treatments consistent with *Āyurveda*. The practice of *Āyurveda* is considered a subsection or branch of the *Atharva Veda*.

But long before this, according to legend, human suffering was the impetus that created the seed of *Āyurveda* on Earth. With the birth of agriculture in India, ten thousand or more years ago, sedentary civilizations developed. As populations grew and lives moved within closer confines, the health of all creatures declined. In response, the infinite wisdom of *Āyurveda* manifested in the mind of the Creator, known in the Hindu religion as *Brahmā*. Lord *Brahmā* shared his divine idea with a few other gods who in turn transmitted it to Lord *Indra*, the king of the Hindu deities and master of the heavenly sphere. Lord *Indra* taught it to sage *Bhāradvāja*, who passed it on to *Atreya Punarvasu*. Atreya's disciple *Agnivesa* is believed to have compiled the work subsequently adapted by the sages *Charaka* and *Drdhabala*, known today as the *Charaka Samhitā*, and established it on Earth for the good of all creatures.

To really know the universe and to know human beings, these sages, or *rishis*, didn't look down microscopes and divide the body into parts. Instead, they experienced the whole human being and the unity of existence. To know life, and how to heal it, the *rishis* embodied Mother Nature as their laboratory of *Āyurveda*. They dissolved into her skies, melted into the sun and stars, and surrendered to the luminous moon. In deep repose, the *rishis* listened to the pulse of the universe, feeling its vibrations in their own. Through observation, intuition, and practical experience, these immortal physicians understood *Āyurveda* and conveyed it to humanity.

Arguably the world's most long-lived system of healing, *Āyurveda* developed in an era when teachings were communicated by mouth; through poetic songs and verses and wise instruction, traditionally from *guru* to student, and later from father-to-son, the knowledge of *Āyurveda* was transmitted and understood. Initially, recording information in hard copy was considered an inferior record-keeping method that rendered knowledge static, cumbersome, and open to misinterpretation. However, as written record-keeping gained ease and favor, the wisdom and practice of *Āyurveda* was documented in the volumes of the *Charaka Samhitā* which today remain the primary texts in the formal study of *Āyurveda*. The *Charaka Samhitā* provides teachings on the fundamental principles governing the maintenance of health and longevity, and prevention and cure of illness. Its teachings offer objective measures of clinical examination; extensive descriptions of the cause, development, diagnosis, forecast, and treatment of many diseases; how to collect, prepare, and apply medicinal plants; the attributes and effects of many foods and drinks on the human body; and medical ethics.

No doubt over time the system of *Āyurveda* influenced (and was influenced by) Buddhist, Jain, Tibetan, Moslem, Chinese, Egyptian, and other medical philosophies, including the Greek system of medicine that began with Hippocrates, and was overthrown by the modern Western medical system only a couple of hundred years ago.

While the wisdom of *Āyurveda* has endured, the path hasn't always been smooth. Around eight hundred years back, Arab Moslem invaders entered the Indian subcontinent and established several Islamic states. Under Mughal rule, the practice of *Āyurveda* was forcefully replaced with *unani*, the Islamic healing system. For five hundred years the practice of *Āyurveda* was punishable by death or limb removal, yet the tradition lived on. As the reign of the Mughals receded, *Āyurveda* slowly returned to the fore. A few hundred years later India was again invaded, this time by the British hierarchy. Again, orders came to close all Ayurvedic schools and, once more on home-soil, the practice of *Āyurveda* became an illegal, punishable offense. It was only seventy years ago, with the reestablishment of Indian independence, that the knowledge and practice of *Āyurveda* resurfaced and was allowed to be practiced openly. Today, after much rebuilding, and with support of the Indian government, the practice of *Āyurveda* continues alongside a Westernized medical system, as well as homeopathy, naturopathy, *unani*, and yoga.

Ayurvedic doctors or *vaidyas* must complete a five-and-a-half-year degree, and some also complete a degree in medicine. For Ayurvedic practitioners modes of study and internship vary.

Of the three main Ayurvedic health strategies—including the administration of herbs, and oil and heat treatments; food and dietary therapies; and activities of the lifestyle or daily routine—medical therapies are available in some dedicated hospitals and also in conjunction with mainstream therapeutic approaches. All three health strategies hold equal importance, predictably overlap, and support the other two. In particular, food and dietary habits are inseparable from our daily lifestyle, and underpin the success (or failure) of all medical and herbal treatments.

In Chapter 1, the first health principle we explore is the importance of living in accordance with the wisdom and cycles of Mother Nature. The next principle, in Chapter 2, is the unique concept of the three *dosha*— *vāta*, *pitta*, and *kapha*— and the value of understanding our unique constitution. In Chapter 3 we examine the prime import of digestion in adequately nourishing the body and supporting every aspect of health. Chapter 4 introduces *Āyurveda's* central healing tenets of *like attracts like* and *opposites reduce*, and focuses on key nutritional principles that make food medicine and balance our unique *dosha* mix. Chapter 5 delves into the principle of eating with awareness and expanding our food relations. And Chapter 6 explores two key food qualities, *langhana* and *brimhana*, the reducing and building nature of foods.

CHAPTER 1

Embrace Mother Nature

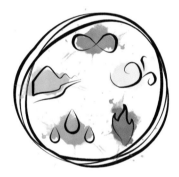

The five great elements

According to *Āyurveda*, Mother Nature is the divine feminine principle of creation, a profound metaphysical origin pertaining to all material existence, to be revered and understood. In Sanskrit, Mother Nature is known as *Prakriti*, literally meaning "that which brings forth." All physical life is seen to emanate from the interplay of Mother Nature's forces. She is the divine mother from whose womb all material creation

flows; all-giving, all-inclusive, ever-present. With her comforting cycles, exquisite self-regulating tendencies, and dynamic equilibrium, she is the first and finest example of balance. If only we were more like our Mother!

Rather than a medical system, at heart *Āyurveda* is a life-positive approach that promotes good health through living in harmony with Mother Nature, of whom we are a part. By observing universal laws and interdependent relationships beyond our seemingly individual existence, and aligning our actions and interests with hers, we harmonize our own nature. Attuning with Mother Nature, including her five great elements, universal qualities, and seasons and cycles, we better understand ourselves and the effects of our actions, and are better equipped to make conscious choices that bear sweeter fruit. Through the foundation of Mother Nature, *Āyurveda* assists us to balance ourselves, and in doing so we act as a balancing force for those around us and our environment.

Five Element Theory

Before modern science reduced life into ever smaller fragments such as nutrients and atoms, many civilizations, including the ancient Indians, then the Greeks acknowledged five great elements of the natural realm—five states of material existence and building blocks of all earthly matter. These five fundamental elements are: earth, water, fire, air, and ether. All physical form, including the human body, are made up of varying combinations of these elements. How does each human come by these substances? Through our father's sperm and mother's ovum that begin physical life; the season and conditions inside the uterus; our mother's nutrition while we are gestating; and every day after birth through eating, drinking,

breathing, and living. In particular, the physical body, or food body, is built and maintained by food. And all food has its unique mix of these elements that become our own flesh and blood. Every day, our habits do much to determine the proportion of these five elements in our system.

In every body, all five elements coexist. Ether is the most rarefied of the five, and acts as the unified space within which all other elements and processes occur. Air, as wind, is the bellows of life that moves all processes along. Fire is the essential element behind digestion and transformation, and the provider of warmth and light. Water, relatively heavy, cool, and liquid adheres the body together. Without water, we dry up and disperse like dust. And earth, the heaviest and most solid substance, provides stability and form.

For *Āyurveda*, the five great elements are a way of describing reality. They are principles by which we can organize and understand the wider world, our own physical body, and how the foods we eat can help or harm us. From the most subtle to the most solid let's get acquainted with their qualities and functions.

Ether (Space)

Conceive ether as a vast field of space; a void that is nonetheless full. Much more than hollowness,

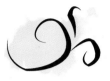

ether is a principle of pervasiveness. An ever-present, formless, cohesive field in which all elements are expressed and contained. Ether is dominated by qualities including subtlety, porosity, softness, light, lack of resistance, and extension. The concept of ether relates to quantum physics' confirmation that everything is created and exists within a pervasive, unified field.

We might think we understand emptiness, but life in built-up environments focuses on objects; we see little horizon or sky. In the physical body, ether dominates in the cavities of the ears, mouth, and nose; the air sacs of the lung; the passage of the small and large intestine; and when empty, the stomach, uterus, and bladder. The hollower the space, the more it vibrates. Ether is associated with sound, and is the element that produces the sense of hearing.

Physical, mental, and spiritual growth and freedom all need the element of space. However, too much space, without a strong Earth connection, creates imbalance through dispersion, drying, and cooling. Excess ether diffuses the body and mind, and fosters restlessness, anxieties, fears, and feelings of emptiness and isolation.

Air (Wind)

Air is rarely unchanging; conveyed by impulse and vibration, its nature is to move. Across the planet, and in the physical body, wind makes movement happen. On Earth, winds search for gaps to fill, moving through crevices, helping mold valleys and canyons. Mighty winds generate dryness and hardness, kindle fire, and bring plants and animals to their knees. At home on a gentle spring day we enjoy a light, spontaneous breeze. Cooling winds blow through open windows; strong gusts flutter the curtains and lift the edge of the rug. We see wind when dust fills the air and leaves dance in trees. We feel wind's movement through the sense of touch. Air is the material cause of our sense of feeling. The attributes of air and ether are similar. Air is cold, dry, light, subtle, rough, mobile, and clear. These two elements spend much time together, and make a powerful combination.

Air is the principle of movement; in the physical body *Āyurveda* sees all movement as driven by the subtle energy of air—the flow of blood and nerve impulses, the digestive fires, all cycles that ensue. The air and *prāna* we breathe in circulate throughout the physical and subtle bodies. Without enough air or *prāna*, vital movements in the body are stifled, earth and water stagnate, fires go out, and *dosha* become imbalanced. Too much air also creates imbalance. In the gut, the gassy air element brings on abdominal cramping, bloating, variable digestion, and an irritable bowel. Too much wind results in constipation and emaciation. As tissues dry out, existing unease intensifies, and new problems occur.

In the mind, the impulse of air carries thoughts and desires. Air feeds mental clarity and vitality and takes joy to flight, yet, air's dryness and coldness can also nurture contraction, fatigue, and desolation. Excess or unwieldy wind conjures nervousness, fears, insomnia, sensitive hearing, excessive speech, and mental hyperactivity.

Fire

For Mother Earth, the sun is the source of all fire, warmth, and light. The sun governs blossoming, ripening, and decay; a principle of transformation and change. All plants and animals pay homage to the sun. Watch the

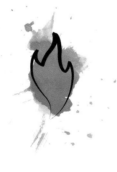

daily unfolding of the flower; the basking lizard; the solar rituals of traditional cultures. Today we can offer the sun homage through the yoga practice of *surya namaskar*. Or simply by being awake and present to the sunrise, absorbing the first blush of morning. Fire is dominated by the qualities of heat, light, radiance, sharpness, subtlety, drying, softening, upward motion, and the ability to spread.

In the food body, fire dominates the entire process of digestion, the constant transformation of the five elements. Fire kindles hunger, and appetite for food, fluids, and sex. So as not to burn us, all digestive fires (such as bodily enzymes) are held in liquid medium. Red blood cells hold heat and are circulated in fluid. Fire is also a principle of radiance. The sense of vision is associated with fire; eyes express shine, luminosity, and color.

For the planet, the loss of the sun's fire would mean global freezing, darkness, and death. And too much heat—the more immediate scenario—will dry us out and burn us up. In the physical body, insufficient fire stunts and slows down, while too much scalds and scorches. Many modern discomforts relate to imbalanced and excess fire, such as symptoms of high blood pressure, fever, heartburn, acid reflux, ulcers, colitis, liver issues, urinary tract infections, skin rashes, inflammations, diarrhea, and excessive thirst and hunger.

In the mind, fire's transforming light graces us with attention, recognition, and understanding, while too much fire ignites frustration, irritability, hot temper, overambition, jealousy, anger, and aggression. On the spiritual path the fire element burns away attachments and illuminates consciousness.

Water

Within our solar system, planet Earth is distinctive in its abundance of water that enables and sustains fecund life. Water is a life-giv-

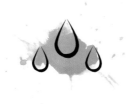

ing, cohering, unifying element that connects molecules together. The qualities of water include liquidity, coolness, wetness, softness, and heaviness. Through its persistent flow, water is inherently strong; in time it can remove all obstacles and seep into every space.

All elements are constantly transformed and recycled, but water particularly so. Today a cloud, tomorrow rain, the day after an ocean or river—only

to condense and rise heavenward again. While the focus of global warming has been on rising levels of carbon dioxide, experts now understand that the process by which Mother Nature regulates heat and climate is through the flow of water. The hydrological cycle is managed by greenhouse water vapor, with each molecule taking on some heat. Evaporation of water from the Earth's surface also allows latent heat to be radiated back to space. And the coalescence of water vapor into clouds reflects the sun's heat, then cools and rehydrates the Earth through droplets of rain.[2]

So too, water constantly cycles through us, providing a vehicle for cooling and quenching, transporting and cleansing. Salt water covers around three quarters of the Earth's surface, and salty water makes up around three quarters of our physical bulk. And both of these mediums are becoming increasingly acidic, clogged with toxins, and less hospitable to life. In the physical body, water forms the basis of plasma, blood, cerebrospinal fluid, mucus, saliva, reproductive fluids, urine, and sweat. Water carries and enables the sense of taste. In the mind, cool, serene water nurtures compassion, sweetness, and love, and melts away hard, stagnating emotions to restore sensitivity and flow.

On Earth, the moon oversees water. As entire oceans sway in response to the moon's cycles, the water within our system also rises and falls. In landscapes, too much water causes floods and overflows. In the body, too much water is experienced as swelling in the ankles or joints; a dull, heavy digestion; excess phlegm or saliva; congested lungs and difficulty breathing; weight gain; and excessive sweating or coldness. On Earth and in the human body, lack of water makes matter dry, hard, and rough; constricting, blocking, and stagnating. Lack of fluidity encourages the growth of cysts, and creates space for air and fire to thrive. Water is the basis of life's juice or sap. Without constant access to clean water, most worldly life would cease. Of all planetary resources, fresh water is arguably most precious.

Earth

Of the five foundational substances, earth is the densest and can be conceived as any firm substance that has structure. In Mother Nature, the solidity of 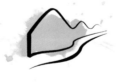 earth is experienced in mountains, soils, shelters, and most foods. In the physical body, earth augments all tissues including bones, teeth, muscles, sinews, skin, hair, and nails, and provides strength, stamina, and stability. We experience the earth element through qualities such as hardness, heaviness, denseness, firmness, thickness, and roughness. Odors are recognized by the nose, our most solid sense organ, which has a special affinity with earth.

As the densest element, earth embodies the principle of inertia—a slowing down of force. The earth element is an ideal ingredient and platform for material creation and physical growth. In the body, too little earth element allows the air, fire, and water elements to blow, burn, wash away, or clog the earth, while too much earth accumulates as tissues, fills spaces, traps water, fire, and air, and slows us down. As well as in the body's channels, we also collect excess earth element though houses, cars, jewels, and gadgets that create baggage and inertia. In the mind, too much earth promotes dullness, attachment, greed, and depression; but in balance the earth element consolidates patience, forgiveness, forbearance, and memory. Balanced "earthy" people promote love, nurturing, and grounding.

Twenty Universal Qualities

To best understand the elements—in our own body, the foods we eat, and in the external environment—*Āyurveda* focuses on the qualities that each element contains. Getting to know the food body, foods and nutrition, and the environment is based on observing the qualities inherent in them. The *rishis* that perceived *Āyurveda*

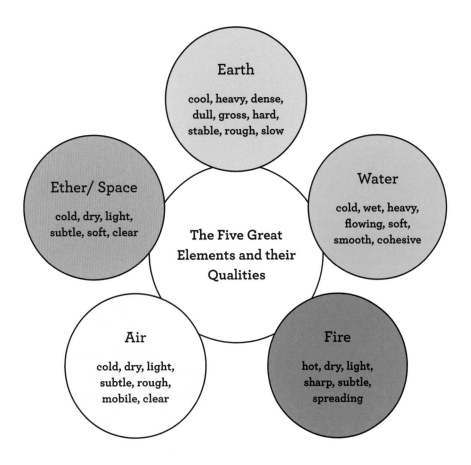

Earth

cool, heavy, dense, dull, gross, hard, stable, rough, slow

Water

cold, wet, heavy, flowing, soft, smooth, cohesive

Ether/ Space

cold, dry, light, subtle, soft, clear

The Five Great Elements and their Qualities

Air

cold, dry, light, subtle, rough, mobile, clear

Fire

hot, dry, light, sharp, subtle, spreading

observed twenty primary qualities shared among the five elements and common throughout life. These twenty key qualities exist as ten pairs that are opposite, but not in opposition:

Cold	Hot
Oily/Moist	Dry
Heavy	Light
Low/Slow/Dull	Sharp/Penetrating
Big/Gross	Small/Subtle
Dense	Flowing/Spreading
Static/Stable	Mobile
Soft	Hard
Smooth	Rough
Cloudy	Clear

In nature, the elements are always mixed up, but each element contains distinct qualities that offer clues to the dominant elements in us. As a working model, each quality exists along a continuum. But not *good* to *bad* or *positive* to *negative*. The twenty qualities are independent of value judgements. Each quality is purely descriptive, ranging from neutral to excessive. And the use of qualities is by no means limited to these twenty. All qualities are useful, but some can be given more importance than others. In foods and in the human body, the qualities of *hot* and *cold*, *oily/moist* and *dry*, and *heavy* and *light* are readily seen or experienced. Qualities of freshness and taste are also fundamental, and will be explored in due course.

Respect Cycles and Seasons

Like the planets and the moon, Earth is a sphere that moves in a circle governed by cycles. Through every phase, the wheel ever turning, sooner or later the Earth completes each full round. Every day-night cycle the Earth revolves on its axis; every year Mother Earth revolves around the sun, bringing the continual cycle of seasons. Eternal cycles exemplify the ebb and flow of life; continual death and renewal. For many native traditions, including the Australian Aboriginals, Mayans, and Aztecs, circular time is central to ecological and spiritual visions. Respecting and paying homage to natural cycles ensures continuation of life. Hindu scriptures also speak of a cycle of ages, in which an era of light and wisdom gives way to times of relative darkness and ignorance, followed again by an age of light.[1]

As a child, the quotidian day-night rotation is an early cyclic experience. The rhythmic pulsing

---

1   This cosmic cycle is known as the *yugas*, a 24,000-year cycle that moves through four stages: *kali yuga* (the dark age), *dwapara yuga*, *treta yuga*, and *satya yuga* (the age of enlightenment). According to this theory, we recently moved from *kali yuga* into *dwapara yuga*, a 2400-year period when man begins to move away from ignorance, and develops electrical and energy devices. During the 4800 years of *satya yuga*, man's wisdom is completely developed, and he works in harmony with the divine plan.

of sun and moon brings heat and cool, dry and moist, action and inaction. The sun and moon act as celestial beats for biological processes including eating, digesting, sleeping, and waste disposal. By the moon's cycling, the menstrual cycle naturally occurs. (Prior to electricity and bright lighting, women ovulated during the full moon, and menstruated in the new moon's dark.) Then there's the rotation of the seasons, and the larger cycle of life. Natural cycles are intrinsic within us, and only need our attention to reawaken. From a health and nutrition perspective, the life cycle, seasonal cycling, and the digestive cycle are particularly important. Let's consider these now.

The Life Cycle
Human life evolves in three main phases. Childhood—from birth to around eighteen years; adulthood—from eighteen to around sixty; and the later years—from sixty until death. In youth, the earth and water elements dominate, and the food body is plumper and moister. In balance, this offers a freshness and disease resistance; in imbalance, children and adolescents are more vulnerable to congestions, especially of the ears, chest, and nose.

In the adult years, the fire element becomes more dominant. This is the period when passions burn strongest and we strive to make our mark. As adults, we are more vulnerable to inflammatory and blood diseases, including disorders of the heart.

In the later years, air and ether dominate, and dry, light qualities take over. The tissues turn rough and brittle, and the mind becomes more diffuse. Over these years, all *dosha* types naturally take on more of these qualities. The life cycle is the broader backdrop against which our innate *dosha* type, and the everyday elements and qualities that influence us, unfold.

Seasonal Cycling
As we rotate around the sun, the slight tilt of the Earth's axis triggers cycles of heat and cold, wet and dry, dark and light. In India and other places of changeable weather, traditional views often note six annual seasons. Closer to the equator, the climate is more stable, and wet and dry seasons offer distinction. In areas closer to the poles, four main seasons tend to dominate, and often change quickly. Land elevation and proximity to water also affect the onset, duration, and intensity of seasons, as have recent population and ecological changes, and global warming.

From an Ayurvedic perspective, the seasonal cycles (all cycles, in fact) revolve according to the dominance of the five great elements. As the Earth rotates, its proximity to the sun's fire, and relative buildup and dispersal of earth, water, fire, and air determine which qualities manifest new seasons, and bring seasons to fruition. In general, summers are dominated by heat, sharpness, and light. In fall, air and winds rule that are mobile, rough, and dry. Cold winters can be sharp and clear; or wet, dull, heavy, and cloudy. Spring, a time of growth and rejuvenation, is warm, moist, and light.

As the elements and qualities in the cosmos change, they naturally affect the physical body. Today however, we insulate ourselves against nature's elements in controlled atmospheres and microclimates. When hot we switch on air conditioning; against cold, we employ central heating. These technologies shield us from the discomfort of extremes, yet form false environments that disorganize natural cycles, and further detach us from Mother Nature.

One foundation of Ayurvedic nutrition is to pay attention to, and work with, our surroundings. Begin to pay attention to the elements and qualities dominating each season, and how over time these factors change. Observe how these dominant elements and qualities influence the physical body. Also notice or investigate which fruits and vegetables grow in different seasons. We return to these ideas, and learn to work with the seasons and *doshas* in Part II on page 109.

The Digestive Cycle

Another cycle worth paying attention to is the daily digestive cycle. While appetite and hunger vary between individuals (according to *dosha* type and other factors), our ability to digest food changes predictably every day. Dawn until mid-morning, 6:00 a.m. to 10:00 a.m., earth and water elements dominate, and it's the body's time to cleanse. From 10:00 a.m. to 2:00 p.m., fire rules, and the digestive fires are strongest while the sun is at its peak. From 2:00 p.m. to 6:00 p.m. winds often increase, and the digestive fires weaken as the day and body cool. Overnight while we fast, the upper gut rests and regenerates, and the lower gut, the colon, accepts and processes metabolic by-products and waste, moving them into channels for elimination at dawn. While we sleep, to maintain healthy function, the entire physical system including the nerves and brain undergo cleansing and rejuvenation.

The daily digestive cycle is also influenced by seasonal cycles. A hot environment pulls the body's heat to the surface, weakening the central digestion. For this reason, cuisines of the tropics tend to favor pungent chilies, returning fire to the belly. In contrast, cold weather drives the digestive fires deeper, strengthening the digestive capacity. In winter, we may comfortably digest heavy meals that trigger indigestion in summer.

According to *Āyurveda*, life on Earth is dominated by five great elements, a range of qualities, a continuous revolution of digestive and seasonal cycles, and the larger cycle of life. By observing and working with Mother Nature we reawaken intrinsic memories and can create daily and seasonal routines that support our natural strengths, complement our personal circumstances and surroundings, and naturally move us toward greater balance and freedom. Chapter 7 on page 109 further embraces Mother Nature, exploring how to function within her daily and seasonal cycles. And in Chapters 6 and 10 on pages 101 and 159, we explore how to truly embody eating.

CHAPTER 2

Get to Know Your Dosha (Constitution)

This chapter looks in-depth at the concept of *dosha*, and the three *dosha*—*vāta*, *pitta*, and *kapha*. Through completing a survey, you will work out which *dosha(s)* dominate in you, then explore the characteristics of each *dosha* type in detail. Lastly, we construct ideas of what balanced *doshas* look like, and consider traits and symptoms that indicate imbalance.

In the human body the *doshas* are not readily seen, touched, or quantified; they are neither food, nor waste, nor physical tissue. Existing in subtle form, the three *doshas* are intelligent biological forces that judiciously manage all levels of growth, function, and structure in the human body. In the creation of life, the subtle forces of *dosha* exist before physical matter.[3] Within the developing fetus, the

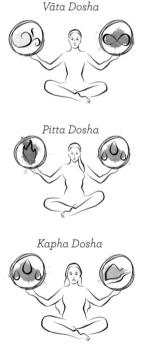

Vāta Dosha

Pitta Dosha

Kapha Dosha

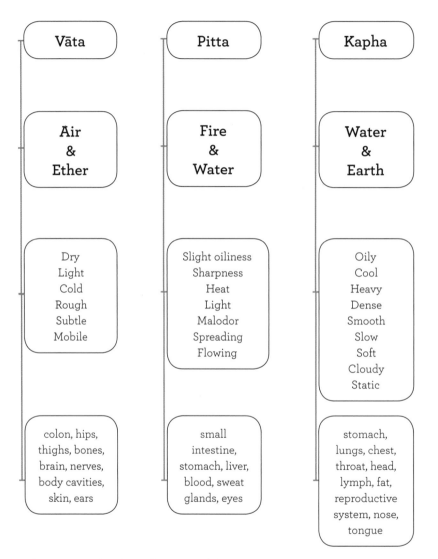

Vāta	Pitta	Kapha
Air & Ether	Fire & Water	Water & Earth
Dry Light Cold Rough Subtle Mobile	Slight oiliness Sharpness Heat Light Malodor Spreading Flowing	Oily Cool Heavy Dense Smooth Slow Soft Cloudy Static
colon, hips, thighs, bones, brain, nerves, body cavities, skin, ears	small intestine, stomach, liver, blood, sweat glands, eyes	stomach, lungs, chest, throat, head, lymph, fat, reproductive system, nose, tongue

The elements and qualities inherent in each dosha, and their main bodily location doshas are the potency that manifest the physical form, and govern it throughout life.

At conception, the relative proportions of the five present elements, largely decide which one or more of the three *doshas* will dominate in our constitution. If the elements of air or ether are strong, *vāta* dominates. If fire rules, *pitta* prevails. If the earth and water elements are dominant, then *kapha dosha* is primary. Each *dosha* manages two of the five great elements. The mix of elements within each *dosha* manifests its particular characteristics and qualities.

In the list of innate qualities, stronger qualities come first. Thus, the strongest expressions of *vāta dosha* are dryness, lightness, and coldness. The most dominant attributes of *pitta dosha* are slight oiliness, sharpness, and heat. In *kapha dosha* the governing qualities are oiliness, coolness, and heaviness. The main location of *vāta dosha* is the colon, of *pitta dosha* is the small intestine, and of *kapha dosha* is the stomach.

When all three *doshas* work together harmoniously in their natural state they support intelligence, vitality, and balance. However, when aggravated or imbalanced, the *doshas* underlie the onset of physical disease. From Sanskrit, the term *dosha* is often translated as "that which is stained," or "that which has fault." Although we are generally born in perfect balance, everyday strains and stresses, and ignorant thoughts and actions, introduce *dosha* imbalance. This flawed functioning corrupts or stains our harmonious nature. If not balanced within the body, the *doshas* become pathogenic factors of disease.

Because the *doshas* are foremost in the creation of the physical body, and also the foremost cause of physical disease, attempts to heal the food body while ignoring the astute guidance system of the *dosha* are bound for a degree of failure. By becoming aware of the *doshas*, particularly our own unique mix, we can work with our metabolic nature, rather than so often against it.

The Sanskrit term *Prakriti* refers to Mother Nature, the essential creative material nature of the universe. At the personal level, *prakriti* refers to the essential nature inherent in each of us, from which all physical creation takes place. In practical terms, our *prakriti* is determined by the mix of elements present at the moment of our conception. This mix of elements represents our most natural, harmonious state. For this reason, our *prakriti* is synonymous with our own perfect health balance.

Once created, our *prakriti* remains essentially unchanged through life (although may be impressionable while we are in the womb and during early childhood, and is influenced by the life cycle). Once formed, our *dosha prakriti*—our unique combination of elements—influences our physical characteristics, metabolic tendencies, and lifelong physical health. As the body contains the mind, our innate constitution also influences how we sense the world, how we think, and traits of personality and temperament. As we shall soon see, those born with a dominance of *vāta's* air, for example, are more prone to dryness, thinness, constipation, and physical and mental mobility. Those dominant in *pitta's* fire element tend to be warm-blooded, intolerant of heat, and more prone to diarrhea and hot tempers. If *kapha's* cool water and earth predominate, tendencies include a sturdy physique, plumpness, congestive illness, and physical and emotional attachments.

We are born with certain elements dominant, and a subtle *dosha* mix, yet during life we accumulate new elements and qualities. If they are complementary, we thrive. If they imbalance our constitution, they make us sick. Most often it's the elements dominating at birth that are the elements that become excessive. Especially as imbalance sets in, we are most likely to accumulate more of the elements we already have. By working with our own unique *dosha* mix, *Āyurveda* provides

an excellent method to understand our physical and mental tendencies, abilities, affinities, strengths, and weaknesses to support health balance.

Diagnose Your Unique Constitution

As *prakriti* is our inborn elemental nature, it is generally revealed by lifelong patterns and tendencies. Yet, throughout life, external destabilizing factors and self-caused influences often take their toll. Over time we take on more elements and qualities, and *dosha* imbalance occurs. Fast forward to now, and often we have lived with imbalance so long that our true nature is simply forgotten. The state of imbalance that covers our true nature is known as *vikriti*, literally meaning "that which covers the *prakriti*." As *prakriti* often becomes somewhat lost or obscured, identifying our lifetime constitution is not always immediately possible. In the short-term, determining our imbalance—the *dosha* that covers our nature—can be more applicable to immediate health.

Accordingly, the following questionnaire has two columns—one for lifetime tendencies (*prakriti*), and one for present tendencies (*vikriti*). For each question, place a letter in *both columns* depending on your option—V (for *vāta*), P (for *pitta*), or K (for *kapha*). For example, in the category "body weight," choose "P" for "Lifetime," if as a child and in general, you have been of average weight. And choose "K" for "Present" if you have gained weight recently, or since youth or middle age. Reflect carefully in order to see yourself as you are, not as you might like to be. If you are unsure of any response, choose whichever feels most correct, or choose "V" for *vāta* if your experience is variable or irregular. Once finished, total up the Vs, Ps, and Ks in both columns.

Diagnose your Birth Constitution (*Prakriti*) and Present Dominant Dosha (*Vikriti*)

CATEGORY	LIFETIME	PRESENT
Body Frame		
V—tall or short, thin, poorly developed physique P—medium height, moderately developed physique K—stout, stocky, big, well-developed physique		
Body Weight		
V—light; it's hard to hold weight P—moderate weight; relatively stable K—heavy; gains weight easily		
Skin Texture		
V—dry, rough or cracked; prominent veins P—moist, pink, freckles, and moles K—white, moist, plump, soft		
Skin Temperature		
V—cold P—warm K—cool		
Hair Quality		
V—coarse, dry, split ends P—fine, soft; grayed or went bald early K—abundant, oily, thick, lustrous		

CATEGORY	LIFETIME	PRESENT
Face Shape		
V—small, thin, long P—medium sized, oval K—large, round, chubby		
Teeth		
V—crooked or erratically placed or spaced P—medium sized, possibly yellowed K—large, even, white		
Gums		
V—dark, receding P—red, soft, bleed easily K—plump and pink		
Tongue Width		
V—narrower than teeth, long and thin P—same width as teeth, oval shaped tip K—wider than teeth, thick, rounded tip		
Quality of Hands		
V—fine, dry, cold; long fingers P—symmetrical, pink, warm K—large, thick; can have short, stubby fingers		
Finger Nails		
V—thin, rough, fissured, cracked, darkened P—strong, pinkish K—thick, smooth, pale		
Appetite		
V—variable, erratic P—strong; can be sharp K—constant, mild		

CATEGORY	LIFETIME	PRESENT
Digestive Strength		
V—variable or weak; can have food allergies P—strong ability to digest K—slow or medium, but steady		
Digestive Disturbances		
V—intestinal gas and windy cramping P—acidity and burning K—feelings of bloating, heaviness, nausea		
Food Attractions		
V—dry, salty, crispy snack foods P—spicy, salty, hot K—sweet, creamy, cold		
Hunger		
V—variable – may binge, snack, or forget to eat P—strong – likes regular, plentiful meals K—little – but may think of food, and enjoys eating		
Food Sensitivities		
V—bean and cabbage families P—onions, tomatoes, fried foods K—dairy, salt, sugar		
Urination		
V—smaller quantity, around two to four times per day P—good quantity four to six times per day, or more K—moderate quantity, around three to five times per day		
Stool		
V—dry, hard, difficult or painful, tends toward constipation P—abundant, loose, sometimes yellowish, tends toward diarrhea K—moderate, solid, sometimes pale, can harbor mucus		

CATEGORY	LIFETIME	PRESENT
Sweat and Body Odor		
V—little, with no smell P—profuse, hot, strongly odious K—moderate, smells sweet or neutral		
Blood Circulation		
V—poor, variable; cold hands and feet P—good circulation; warm hands and feet K—slow but steady; cool hands and feet		
General Activities		
V—quick, fast, erratic, hyperactive P—motivated, purposeful, goal-seeking K—slow, steady, methodical		
Strength and Endurance		
V—poor endurance; starts and stops P—moderate endurance K—slow in starting, but good endurance		
Sensitivity to Environment		
V—dislikes cold, wind; sensitive to dryness; seeks warmth P—dislikes heat and direct sun; prefers shade and coolness K—dislikes cold, damp weather; doesn't mind wind or sun		
Disease Tendencies		
V—nervous system issues, pain, mental unrest, insomnia, disordered eating, arthritis P—fevers, inflammations, infections, ulcers, high blood pressure, heart attack K—respiratory system diseases, mucus, edema, weight gain, cysts, and tumors		
Resistance to Disease		
V—poor, variable; weak immune system P—medium K—good, consistent; immunity can be strong		

CATEGORY	LIFETIME	PRESENT
Mental Nature		
V—quick, adaptable, indecisive, impulsive P—factual, penetrating, critical K—slow, steady, calm		
Speech Habits		
V—quick, talkative, inconsistent, erratic P—moderate, argumentative, convincing K—slow, concise; not so talkative		
Emotional Response		
V—quick, but soon over P—hot, irritated, defensive K—slower, can be more caring, but can also hold a grudge		
Emotional Tendencies		
V—anxiety, fears, nervousness, too many worries; if depressed, it passes P—frustration, irritability, anger, jealousy, willfulness K—calm, sentimental, attached; if depressed, it's heavy		
Relationship to Objects		
V—they are not very important, but can sometimes buy a lot P—they are important, purposeful; fulfill personal functions K—they are practical and provide comfort		
Relationship to Money		
V—it's not very important; spends easily P—it's useful to gain respect or control; spends for a purpose K—it's important to have; spends with difficulty		
Social Relations		
V—relates easily; can be light or superficial P—relates well; can be dominating K—relates with more difficulty; can be loving		

CATEGORY	LIFETIME	PRESENT
Friends		
V—has many, but not deep P—has close or intense relationships K—has few, but very deep		
Love Relationships		
V—tends to have many; can be somewhat erratic P—may marry for position or looks K—one partner, very faithful		
Life Goals		
V—change frequently, not so important P—very important, takes a determined approach K—are fairly fixed for life		
Sleep		
V—light, restless, tends toward insomnia P—moderate, may wake up but sleeps again K—heavy; difficulty waking up in the morning		

Totals:
Record the number of times you wrote V, P, or K in each column.

Lifetime = V_____ P _____ K _____

Present = V_____ P _____ K _____

Having totaled the Vs, Ps, and Ks in each column, the *dosha* with the highest score represents the dominant *dosha* type; the next highest score, the next most prevalent; and the lowest score is the *dosha* least prominent. In your lifetime, or birth constitution, if one *dosha* has numbered markedly higher and is clearly foremost in your constitution, this indicates a "single" or "pure" *dosha*-type. If two *dosha* appear to a similar degree, you probably have a "mixed" or "dual" constitution. This would be indicated, for example, in a score V=17, P=15, and K=5, suggesting a mixed *vāta-pitta* constitution. In this survey, if two *dosha* appear within a range of plus or minus 4 points, a dual-type constitution is probably indicated. A score of V=7, P=10, and K=20 indicates a pure *kapha* type. Another way to conceive your constitution is to rank the relative contributions of each *dosha*. The scores above could be viewed as: V1 P1 K3 and V2 P2 K1, respectively.

In defining *dosha*-type, the purpose is not to classify or pigeonhole. One constitution is not better or worse than another; all have their own attributes and challenges. With new ideas circulating, let's take a closer look at each of the *doshas*, and the three dual-type constitutions— *vāta-pitta, pitta-kapha,* and *kapha-vāta.* The seventh possibility is the tri-*doshic*-type, with equal proportions of all three *doshas* present at birth. This mix confers a great robustness and balance, but is rare, and not explored in detail.

In the *dosha's* three-way relationship as physical managers, *vāta* manages *pitta* and *kapha*. *Vāta* is also most prone to disruption. This makes *vāta dosha* an entity that needs looking after, so *vāta* is where we begin.

On the Move with *Vāta Dosha*

In Sanskrit, the term *vāta* derives from the verb "va," meaning to move or carry. Referring to the wind, *vāta* also translates to "what blows." *Vāta dosha* is an intelligent cosmic force that manages

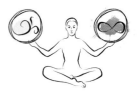

the elements of air and ether. Similar to these two elements, *vāta dosha* has no particular size or physical shape. Invisible to the eye, we know *vāta* through its actions and functions. In the body, *vāta* expresses directional movement and all impulses and rhythms. When in balance, the movement of *vāta dosha* provides physical and mental vitality and vigor.

Among the three *doshas*, *vāta* can be labelled the leader for its ability to coordinate and move. When transport is needed, *vāta dosha* springs into action. *Prāna*, breath, food, water, blood, hormones, lymph, wastes, thoughts, speech, emotions, sense reception and expression, and all nerve impulses, move due to *vāta dosha*. In its natural state, *vāta* coordinates all metabolic processes, sensory functions, and communication. The rhythm of tissues and organs is different, yet *vāta* controls all tempos. Cycles in time—the baby becoming the child, adolescent, adult, and elderly citizen—are synchronized by *vāta dosha*. Balanced *vāta* likes regular movement. Neither erratic, nor excessive. And when no movement is necessary, *vāta* holds still.

The "home" of *vāta dosha* in the physical body is the colon. Other important locations include the ears (and sense of hearing), skin (sense of touch), bones, and the nervous tissues, including the brain. These locations can be the first to show signs of *vāta* imbalance. Dry constipation; crackling or ringing ears, balance issues, noise sensitivity; dry, cracked, rough skin; osteoporosis; nervousness, anxiety, and physical or mental stress or debility.

In their physical characteristics, those born with *vāta* dominance tend to be naturally thin-framed, fine-boned, and light in musculature. The dominant qualities of *vāta*—dry, light, cold, rough, and mobile—all promote loss of structure. In the *vāta* physique, bones, joints, tendons or veins can be prominent. *Vāta* individuals may have relatively dark complexions, and darker hair. The eyes, which may also be dark, can be dry, recessed, or twitchy. Growing up under a dominance of air and ether, the teeth of *vāta* types are often crooked and may be large, small, or protruding. Given the tendency of wind to be erratic, the expression of ears, nose, or feet may somehow be irregular (large, small, crooked, or curved). The tongues of those with *vāta* in the birth constitution tend to be long, thin, and mobile, and sometimes curved.

When *vāta* is out of balance and occurs in excess, the cool, dry qualities of air and ether can manifest in cold hands or feet and dull, rough, dry skin, hair, lips, or tongue. In *vāta* excess, internal organs also lack lubrication, resulting in symptoms such as hoarse voice, dry throat, hiccups, burping, muscular stiffness, cracking joints, and arthritis. Digestive issues related to an excess of air and ether include excessive flatulence; bloating; a variable, nervous, sensitive digestion; and constipation. In all types of pain, *vāta* is implicated. Especially pain that is striking or piercing.

As they are cool already, *vāta*-dominant types tend to feel the cold. Fall months that are dry, light, cold, clear, and windy are particularly *vāta* aggravating. When disturbed, and especially in later life, *vāta* types often experience light, scanty sleep, or suffer from insomnia. Due to their delicate state, those with *vāta* dominance may have few or no children. All chronic degenerative diseases, such as arthritis, Parkinson's, and Alzheimer's have roots in excessive *vāta*. When it comes to food and drink, the appetite and thirst of *vāta* types are often variable. Sometimes nibbling; sometimes gorging; other times forgetting to eat. High *vāta* supports food sensitivities and allergies, and often involves bloating and gas.

The light, mobile qualities of *vāta* activate the body, and motivate the mind. *Vāta dosha* brings things to our attention—such as sense impressions, and natural impulses to eat, burp, urinate, defecate, laugh, cry, imagine, and sleep. In balance, *vāta* inspires from within, driving enthusiasm and motivation for life. Existence feels light and free. Sitting idle is a punishment for *vāta*-driven individuals, who prefer action and change. Those with *vāta* constitution can be avid exercisers who, with their somewhat fragile nature, tire easily and risk overdoing it. The mobile nature of *vāta* also manifests through seeking variety in furniture, living location, clothes, partners, and friends. Lack of change brings boredom. Relationships are not necessarily long.

When *vāta* types are in balance, this supports a clear, alert, creative mind. Those *vāta* by birth often do well in inventive fields, and make inspired artists. *Vāta* types have the capacity to make good money, yet have difficulty saving, and often spend frivolously. Those with *vāta* dominance are good at initiating tasks, but may be poor at focusing and completing. Others can see this as fickle or unreliable, but it is only *vāta* expressing its nature. Mentally, *vāta* individuals understand quickly, but can also daydream and be quick to forget. They may possess knowledge, yet lack self-confidence, or be indecisive. But by and large, *vāta's* light, mobile nature creates curious, adaptable, generous, social, joyful human

beings. Those who are anti-conformist and enjoy moving beyond existing boundaries likely have *vāta* in their constitution.

Rather than put their ingenuity to use, too much air and ether manifests as a scatterbrain, spaced-out, or the proverbial chatterbox speaking relentlessly about irrelevant things. Imbalanced *vāta dosha* supports the tendency to hold a negative or changeable self-view, or to be emotionally insecure, or timid. When unsteady, surges of emotion, fear, anxiety, nerves, and phobias (often related to heights or enclosed spaces) can come to the fore. Fragile and imbalanced *vāta* types are prone to experience stress, shock, grief, loneliness, disturbed sleep, nervous breakdowns, and cyclic depression. All depressive states are in some way related to *vāta*. With their light, airy nature, *vāta* types who sit in meditation can experience the blissful void.

Factors that Precipitate *Vāta Dosha* Imbalance

Any environment, food, and lifestyle that involves qualities of coldness, dryness, lightness, roughness, and mobility can increase *vāta dosha*. Exposure to:

· Windy, dry, cold, or erratic weather, especially in fall and late winter, and

during seasonal change. (The dry, light qualities of summer can mildly aggravate *vāta*, but the heat keeps it in check.)
- Dry, light mid-to-late afternoons.
- High altitudes.
- Erratic or heavy exercise.
- All forms of public transport (planes, cars, trains, buses, motorbikes), and moving from one place to another.
- Shocks, traumas, and accidents.
- Excessive colonics and cleansing therapies.

The elements of air and ether also enter us through foods and eating patterns. Including:

- *Dry foods*, such as crackers, dry breakfast cereals, and popcorn. These foods actually take moisture from the body.
- *Drying tastes of pungent, bitter, or astringent foods*. We examine these in detail shortly.
- *Refined foods*, especially flours and sugars with their oils and complexity removed.
- *Overly rough foods*, such as nuts and undercooked legumes, especially if underchewed or overeaten.
- *Frozen foods*, such as processed meals, and fresh meals that have been frozen.

Freezing dries food out and makes it hard to digest.
- *Dehydrated products*, such as powdered milk and mixes, even if reconstituted.
- *Leavened bread*, baked and risen on pockets of yeasted air, is invariably light and dry.
- *Cold food and drinks*, especially in cold seasons and environments.
- *Eating too little food*, or too much deprivation and fasting.
- *Irregular meal patterns*.

In the life cycle, over age sixty is considered the *vāta* stage of life. The elements of air and ether increase, the tissues thin, and the physical body becomes drier. The transition from the middle years through menopause is also innately *vāta* (and *pitta*) aggravating.

Finally, while excessive movement provokes *vāta dosha*, the impediment of movement, including blockage of channels, or suppression of natural urges (such as urinating, defecating, farting, sneezing, burping, yawning, vomiting, eating when hungry, drinking when thirsty, crying when sad, orgasming when aroused, sleeping when fatigued, and breathing on exertion) also irritate *vāta*.

Symptoms of *Vāta Dosha* Imbalance

Many characteristics of *vāta dosha* and *vāta* imbalance have been discussed already. Common signs include dryness or roughness of skin, and internal dryness, experienced as cracking joints, cramping muscles, a rough or cracked tongue, constipation (not opening the bowels daily), and stools that are dry, hard, or rough. A gassy, bloated, erratic elimination (classic symptoms of what is commonly known as irritable bowel) is also associated with *vāta*. As are problems associated with the ears, such as ringing, poor balance or dizziness, and symptoms such as lightheadedness, unsteadiness, feelings of emptiness, floating, or being ungrounded. All nerve issues are related to *vāta*, including tremors, tingling, pulsating, and heartbeat abnormalities, especially fast or erratic. Cutting or splitting pain is another sign, as are emaciation, or unintentional weight loss. Regarding emotions and modes of expression, excessive or uncontrolled communication, excess fears, insecurities, compulsions, and anxiety or panic attacks all point to *vāta* excess.

Firing Up *Pitta Dosha*

The Sanskrit word *pitta* is derived from the root *tapa* which literally means "what cooks." Allied with the elements of fire and water, *pitta* is hot and transformative by nature—the only *dosha*

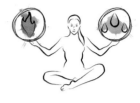

with fire in its mix. In the physical body, the fire element is always suspended in a liquid medium to protect delicate tissues. The marriage of fire and water provides *pitta* its qualities of slight oiliness, sharpness/penetration, heat, light, sour/pungent odor, liquidity, and the tendency to spread.

Around the navel is the chief *pitta* zone, especially the small intestine, liver, gallbladder, lower stomach, pancreas, and spleen. In every human system, *pitta dosha* dominates the process of digestion, food conversion, and assimilation into tissues. As well as digest foods, *pitta* fires kindle metabolic transformations in every living cell. Given their fire predominance, *pitta* types often possess a strong digestion, appetite, and thirst. If *pitta* is excessive, digestion can turn sharp and burning.

The fire of *pitta* also provides heat and maintains bodily warmth. Being naturally hot-blooded, those with *pitta* dominance tend to be intolerant of excess sunlight or heat. As well as the blood cells, the sweat and sebaceous glands also hold and release heat. When *pitta* dominates, the tendency to sweat is increased, often accompanied by yellow stains and a pungent odor. *Pitta* types can produce copious quantities of sweat, urine, and feces.

Regarding physical stature, those with *pitta* constitution can enjoy a moderately robust physique, with medium musculature and frame. When in balance, *pitta* types seldom gain or lose much weight. Through the combination of fire and water, *pitta* and mixed *pitta* types enjoy a soft, supple, shiny complexion that can range from moist and rosy, to flushed red with broken capillaries. *Pitta's* glowing, ruddy complexion can be dotted with freckles and moles. In the hair, a lustrous, luminous quality may be observed. However, many *pitta*-dominant individuals go prematurely bald or gray. Reflecting the sharp quality of fire, *pitta* people can possess angular features such as a pointed chin or nose. Their teeth may also be pointed and yellowing with a tendency toward bleeding gums. *Pitta* tongues are shiny and rosy, of medium thickness and length. The eyes of *pitta* types are often bright, but can be sensitive to light, and the whites are prone to yellow.

In everyone, fire's light, warm, subtle, penetrating qualities influence the way we think. Through subtle *pitta* transformation, ideas and experiences can be digested and understood. Pure and mixed *pitta* types can be blessed with great clarity and wisdom. In the psychology, fire's spreading nature translates to the impulse to be purposeful, goal-oriented, probing, and committed. *Pitta* types can have an incredible eye for detail.

Highly disciplined and determined, *pitta* and *pitta* dual-type individuals are often happiest when striving toward goals that foster a sense of personal or social achievement. Fire's light, spreading qualities can flame social graces and the lucidity of an excellent orator. *Pitta*-dominant types may choose noble professions through which their recognition can spread.

In a balanced state, *pitta* individuals can achieve much. Yet, excess *pitta* can drive pride, and the will to social and material grandeur. If there's money in *pitta's* pocket, it's spent on luxuries, or objects toward betterment. Emotionally balanced *pittas* exude warmth, cheerfulness, and courage. Yet when the fire is excessive, *pitta's* hot, sharp nature is quick to flame; prone to irritability and anger, and critical, self-righteous, and perfectionistic tendencies that kindle jealousy and hate.

Pitta individuals can be strong-willed, but in excess become fanatical or aggressive. Fears of failure or loss-of-control may abound; moods swing from anger to despair. As high achievers, *pitta* types often take on too much. Yet when convinced of the rationale for change, can apply themselves supremely and establish new order. The main danger in seeking transformation is that they try to achieve everything at once.

Factors that Precipitate *Pitta Dosha* Imbalance

Any environment, food, and lifestyle that involve qualities of heat, light, pungency, or drying (which increases heat) can increase *pitta dosha*, such as exposure to:

- Hot sun or weather, especially around midday, and in summer.
- Warm, wet seasons.
- Dry, arid places such as deserts.
- Fires, central heating, and other warming, drying devices.
- Over-exercise, including too much sex.
- Too much competition.
- Excessive hot emotions such as irritation, frustration, jealousy, and anger; overindulgence in almost any emotion is bound to increase *pitta* (and *vāta*).

Pitta's fire element also enters us through our diet, including:

- *Foods and fluids hot in temperature* (especially in warm environments and seasons).
- *Pungent, sour, and salty tastes.* More on this shortly.
- *Dry and dehydrating foods* (these intensify *pitta's* fire).

Symptoms of *Pitta Dosha* Imbalance

Excess *pitta* fire causes a variety of symptoms, all related to excess heat. This includes inflammation (now known to be a primary precursor of many modern-day illnesses and syndromes), high blood pressure, heartburn, hyperacidity, acid reflux, and sour or acidic tastes in the mouth. Ulceration of the mouth, stomach, and gut; acne and spreading rashes; jaundice and liver disorders; stones in the gallbladder and kidneys; and urinary tract infections are all associated with *pitta*. Other signs include burning sensations and fevers; pungent sweat, urine and feces, including hot, often yellowish diarrhea; and yellowness or redness of the whites of the eyes or tongue. In the emotional realm, excessive irritability, frustration, jealousy, anger, and aggression are imbalanced *pitta* traits.

Hanging out with *Kapha Dosha*

From its original Sanskrit, the term *kapha* translates to "what sticks," referring to the nature of earth and water to adhere. In the food body, *kapha* is the intelligent principle that manages the coherence of earth and water into struc-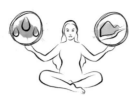ture and form. Bodily lubrication is also *kapha's* domain. The dominance of water and earth creates oily, lubricating, protective substances such as cerebrospinal fluid, synovial fluid, mucus, and lymph. All cellular secretions, mucus membranes, and fatty cushioning exist because of *kapha*. When something needs to be built, oiled, or protected, call in *kapha dosha*.

With its heavy, slow, cool, dense, slimy qualities, the way of *kapha* is augmentation unit-by-unit, cell-by-cell. *Kapha* builds and strengthens tissues and provides the structure in which *vāta* and *pitta* operate, and restrains their light, active, consuming natures. Above the diaphragm is considered the *kapha* zone, foremost the upper stomach, lungs, throat, mouth, tongue, sinuses, nasal passages, and the head in general. All of these structures require ongoing lubrication. *Kapha* also dominates in fatty tissues and the reproductive system.

Balanced *kapha* constitution are blessed with a strong body, well-lubricated joints, plump organs, and excellent physical and mental endurance. *Kapha* dominance cultivates a large physical frame, heavy bones, solid muscles, and well-covered tendons and veins. Plus, a tendency to become overweight, and for weight gain to be difficult to shed. *Kapha* types often have large attractive eyes, strong white teeth, and thick curly hair. The tongue can be short, wide, thick, or immobile, and pale pink in color. Speech may be deep and melodious, and the skin pale, oily, smooth, and cool compared to relations by race or family.

When it comes to eating, *kapha* individuals tend to possess a steady hunger, thirst, and digestion, and can be drawn to sweet and heavy food. As their metabolism is geared toward cohesion and building, these food choices don't bode well. Weight gain is further invited by *kapha's* slow, static nature, and fondness for sitting and sleeping. A comfortable demeanor is a leisurely (some may say sluggish) pace. If too much heaviness exists, *kapha* types experience difficulty initiating activity, but once on the move enjoy physical exertion and a new sense of vitality and freedom. Cool and moist already, mornings can be difficult. With their cloudy, slow qualities, a caffeine fix can be needed to kick-start the day.

In the psychology, *kapha's* steady qualities motivate a desire for permanence and security.

Their social life is often dominated by the same group of people, and *kapha* types seek environments that are comfortable and familiar for themselves and their family. *Kapha* qualities nurture patience and perseverance, but they can be better at finishing than starting. Kapha types often learn slowly, and need repetition, but once learned they never forget. *Kapha* individuals work well in association, and are willing to follow others. With their natural cohesiveness, they make and save money easily.

The natural stability of *kapha* enables one to weather life's storms. Balanced *kapha* dominance supports stillness, peace, deep faith, and grounding. Nurturing, compassionate, loyal, and forgiving, their natural cohesiveness can manifest through physical affection, such as a love of hugging. In relationships, *kapha* types can become deeply attached. Those with *kapha* dominance may avoid conflict and feel compelled to keep the status quo.

Kapha's heavy qualities readily create laziness, passivity, and stagnation. In excess, or if security is threatened, *kaphas* can tend toward greed, attachments, and worldly desires. And in their quest to seek stability, imbalanced *kapha* types can become controlling or manipulative. Imbalanced *kapha* can hold onto old issues, ideas, and attitudes—baggage that burdens the food body, the

vital body, and the mind or mental sheath. When disturbed, a rigid, obstructive mindset devolves that prevents growth and expansion. Overall, however, ancient *Āyurveda* lauds this *dosha* for its plump, robust, grounded merits.

Factors that Precipitate *Kapha Dosha* Imbalance

Environments, foods, and lifestyles involving oiliness, dampness, heaviness, coolness, denseness, softness, stagnancy, or cloudiness increase *kapha dosha*. This means exposure to:

- Wet winter months, early spring, and cool, heavy, damp weather.
- Early morning and late evening when moister, heavier qualities abound.
- Inadequate exercise and physical activity.
- Too much sleep, sleeping into the morning, and naps after eating and during the day.

The elements of earth and water also enter us through foods. Especially detrimental to *kapha* types include:

- *Oily, fatty foods* that introduce moist, heavy qualities, suppress digestion, and encourage tissue gain.

- *Cold, dense foods*, such as dairy products. The cool, cloudy, liquidity of milk and yogurt feed *kapha* directly.
- *Foods that are excessively sweet, salty, or sour.* We will come to these shortly.
- *Drinking too much*, especially cold drinks, and milk.

In general, earth and water are the primary elements that enter us through food. Plus, fluids are secreted in the form of saliva and gastric juices. Thus, every time we eat, and for about the next hour, we naturally support and increase *kapha dosha*.

Symptoms of *Kapha Dosha* Imbalance

Common signs of too much *kapha* earth and water include drowsiness after eating; a heavy, "stuck" digestion; excessive mucus and nose blowing; congestion of the lungs, throat, and sinuses; swollen glands; and repeated phlegmy coughs and colds. With its pension to adhere and accumulation, additional symptoms include edema and fluid retention, cysts and tumors (generally benign), and increasing fatty tissues. Other signs involve light-colored stool, cloudy white urine, and a thick white coating on the tongue. Mentally, feelings of lassitude, lethargy, and drowsiness; excessive sleep; waking without enthusiasm; heavy depression; and

obstructiveness, possessiveness, and greed all point to *kapha* excess.

Mixed Constitutions: When Two *Doshas* Rule

In total, *Āyurveda* recognizes seven distinct constitutions or metabolic types. Three single— or pure-types—*vāta*, *pitta*, and *kapha*. Three dual types—*vāta-pitta* (*pitta-vāta*), *vāta-kapha* (*kapha-vāta*), and *pitta-kapha* (*kapha-pitta*). And one balanced or *tridoshic* type. Both classical and modern experience suggest that mixed-type constitutions are most common. When two *doshas* rule, the qualities of both *doshas* mix and vary in domination. Those with a dual *dosha prakriti* or constitution may follow one or the other more strongly, or be a blend of both *doshas*. Sometimes two *doshas* nurture opposite qualities (such as *vāta* and *kapha*), and can cancel each other out, making diagnosis more difficult. When two *dosha* rule, we need to cultivate respect and understanding of both. Let's examine characteristics and attributes of the three dual-type *dosha*.

Vāta-Pitta (and *Pitta-Vāta*) *Dosha*

Physically, *vāta-pitta* types tend to be of fine-to-medium frame. In balance they are often slim, and if active can develop defined muscles. Their sporty build is a gift to runners, skiers, and athletes. Reflecting their combination, they like to move (*vāta*) and compete (*pitta*). As both air and fire have drying qualities, *pitta-vāta* people must be vigilant against dehydration and overheating.

Those with a combination of *vāta's* mobility and *pitta's* spreading fire harbor good life-energy. Whipped along by *vāta's* wind and *pitta's* transforming fires, *vāta-pitta* types generally enjoy a strong appetite, hunger, and digestion, and love a good meal. In imbalance, digestion can become sharp or irregular, falling prey to acid reflux or gas. In balance, the coldness of *vāta* tempers *pitta's* fires to offer those with *vāta-pitta* constitution good disease resistance. There may be sensitivity to sound or light.

In the psychology, the mingling of wind and fire generate an explosive mix, either fanning the flames of brilliance or fostering red-blooded rage. In their innate qualities, both *dosha* share the attribute of lightness which can fashion creative, adaptable individuals with luminous intelligence. *Vāta-pitta* types can be bright, highly imaginative, venerated thinkers. The *vāta* pension for innovation, and *pitta* persistence and focus, support the creation of dreams and the ability to see them through to concrete form. While pure *vātas* can be chatty, and pure *pittas* not chatty at all, *vāta-pitta* types can be clear, easygoing communicators, successful leaders in business and teaching.

Among their challenges, *vāta-pitta* types can become lost in thought or mentally irritable. They can exhibit nervous qualities or blazing fires or a reactive blend of the two. High levels of stress may elicit a fear response, or anger, bullying, or ascendancy. In imbalance, this combination can exhibit self-assurance or even conceit, but when questioned or censured, be overcome by uncertainty and confusion. Enfeebled *vāta-pitta* types may try to dominate weaker individuals. There can be an inclination to physical and mental addictions.

Because *pitta-vāta* types are naturally less abundant in *kapha*, they can lack stable, earthy qualities, and come to feel ungrounded or unsteady. In pursuit of balance, this dual type functions best in loving, maternal environments. The presence of *kapha*-dominant friends or partners is a blessing.

Pitta-Kapha (and Kapha-Pitta) Dosha
In their physical nature, those with mixed *pitta* and *kapha* constitution benefit from *kapha's* stable, robust attributes, and the warm, moderate qualities of *pitta*. *Pitta-kapha* types can excel at competitive sports and physically demanding activities, and generally benefit from regular

exercise and activity. *Pitta's* strong digestion alongside *kapha's* slow, robust metabolism support good health and longevity.

Both *pitta* and *kapha* constitutions tend to enjoy their food, making this constitution prone to overeating. Overindulgence however, reliably aggravates both *dosha* and promotes weight gain over time. While youthful, the digestion may cope with heavy, fatty foods, but toward middle age, tissues and congestion buildup. The shared water element promotes a natural dampness and oiliness. These individuals can endure temperature extremes and seasonal changes, but may struggle in humid weather. They often do best in dry, temperate zones.

In the mind, the merging of *pitta* drive and intelligence with the stability of *kapha* creates a good foundation for balance. The cool solidity of *kapha* helps to temper the hot fires of *pitta*. This mixed type is not usually a risk-taker, but adjusts well to slow change. Often conservative and routine-oriented, once galvanized, *kapha-pitta* individuals can bring about momentous personal and social change. In business, ambition and passion mix with committed, nurturing qualities to produce worthy executives and managers.

While both *pitta* and *kapha* types can possess a fondness for comforts, when life is too easy, this mixed constitution becomes complacent, conceited, or unhappy. Physical and mental challenges are beneficial for the *pitta-kapha*, who can otherwise have it all their way. In the psychology, the shared element of water can create an oiliness that promotes the sliding of unwanted realities. In this obscured state, *pitta-kapha* individuals may recognize adulation, and ignore unwelcome censure. When imbalanced, this constitution can get caught up in seeking superficial luxuries or substance addictions. Relatively low in air and ether, *pitta-kapha* individuals may need some encouragement to step out of a cozy lifestyle to nurture stronger spiritual connection.

Vāta-Kapha (and Kapha-Vāta) Dosha

As a basic tenet, you could say that *vāta* and *kapha doshas* are two qualitative opposites—fast and slow; variable and fixed; light and heavy. A mix that offers the potential for great characteristics, and also great conflicts. The *vāta* side likes movement, change, and irregularity—to stay up late, and eat all hours. On the other hand, *kapha dosha* prefers stability, and dependable eating and sleeping. The common trait is the quality of cold, as neither contains heat. While this can be a chilly combination, the insulation of *kapha* can shield this dual type from *vāta's* intense freeze.

In physical stature, those with shared *vāta-kapha* dominance can be of moderate build, like *pitta*. Generally speaking, *vāta-kapha* constitutions are strong and resilient to illness. Their nagging issues may be minor aches and pains, constipation, congestions, edema, or weight gain. *Kapha's* congestive qualities can be exacerbated by *vāta's* dryness.

At heart, *kapha-vāta* types can be modest, humble, selfless, kind, and shy. If socially oriented, they are good at relating, and can excel in caring or motherly capacities. With the creativity of *vāta* and stability of *kapha*, they can be far-sighted, and have what it takes to excel in artistic endeavors. Mixed *vāta-kapha* types can be intuitive, and happiest when in touch with Mother Nature.

With their mix of opposing qualities, this dual-type can be somewhat of a chameleon. Emotional depth can be thwarted by changeability. Self-attitudes can alternate from light to heavy, open to closed, spontaneous to rigid. Snappy decisions can be made; other times, fruitless energy is wasted. On important issues, *kapha-vāta* individuals may avoid confrontation, or fail to have their say. The lack of *pitta* fire can induce difficulty integrating the personality. Despite essential solidity and vision, these individuals may feel dissatisfied with life. Ultimately, it is essential that both sides of their nature are acknowledged and comprehended.

Getting to know your unique constitution and the nature of any imbalance takes time. Don't be quick to jump to conclusions. Simply begin to observe. Factors that increase each *dosha* and symptoms of excess *dosha* are important considerations, but are influenced by many dynamics, and are not set in stone. Plus, current imbalances mask our true nature very well. Those who appear of single constitution can realize over time that a second *dosha* also influences their nature; or a seeming dual constitution is really a matter of *dosha* excess. So too, *dosha* decrease and restoration of balance takes time. The ancient Ayurvedic text, *Ashtanga Hridyam*, explains that flood waters gush into the city very fast, but the reversal process is slow. With new knowledge in hand, let's now explore Ayurveda's nutritional healing approach, eating to balance your unique constitution.

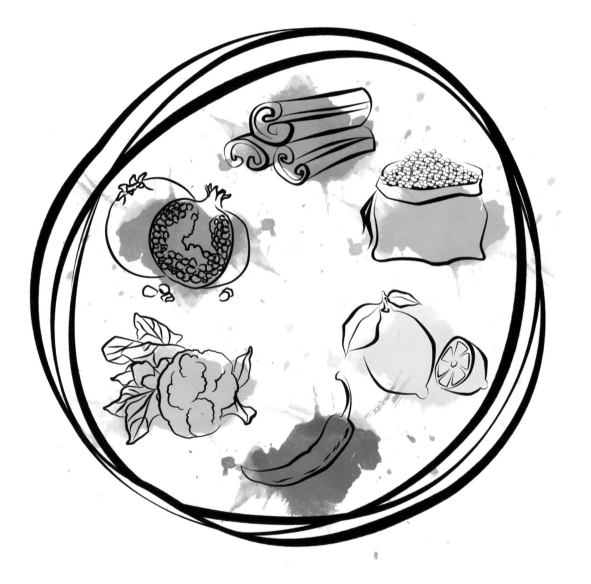

CHAPTER 3

Eat to Balance Your Unique Constitution

For vitality and long life, maintaining the natural balance and rhythm of the *doshas* in the body is *Āyurveda's* primary preventative and therapeutic goal. Working with the *doshas* involves choosing food qualities and tastes, meal times and patterns, quantities, and eating behaviors that complement our unique constitution, within daily and seasonal cycles. This chapter examines how to navigate food and dietary choices to balance your *dosha* type, beginning with the fundamental question: why seek health as balance?

Why balance? Because the natural order of every plant and animal *is* harmony and balance. The Western medical concept of balance is known as

homeostasis, the mechanism by which chemical and functional activities are constantly adjusted to maintain equilibrium of all bodily systems. The concept of homeostatis understands that every part of the body shares responsibility for sustaining itself and coordinating with the whole. Body temperature, electrolyte and acid-base balance, hormone and enzyme parameters, and tissue production require constant regulation and resetting. When interrupted by imbalanced forces, innate inner intelligence seeks realignment. But partial or failed rebalancing results in disease.

According to Eastern beliefs including *Taoism*[2] and traditional Chinese medicine, a balance of

2   *Taoism* is a spiritual philosophy of Chinese origin that emphasizes simplicity, tranquility, and harmonious attunement with natural laws. Its main teachings are in the *Tao te Ching*, written by Lao Tzu over four and half thousand years ago.

the opposing yet complementary forces of *yin* and *yang* underlie all manifest creation. Health is contingent on balancing hot, dynamic, outgoing, masculine *yang* with cool, tranquil, receptive, feminine *yin*. As degrees exist in everything, nothing is wholly *yang* or *yin*. Balance can exist because each polarity holds the opposite deep at its core. However, when one force becomes excessive it dominates and consumes the other. Over recent centuries, the hot, extroverted force of *yang* has burned away cool, nurturing *yin* energies, which desperately need replenishing.

We must also balance the inner and outer. Much ill health exists because we pitch our own destiny against the force of cosmic laws. For *Āyurveda*, balancing the inner with the outer involves working with Mother Nature's natural rhythms and cycles. So too, we must be in contact with the ecosystem, but remain centered at our core. The *Sufi* technique of whirling is a means to find this focus. Slowly as the body spins the whirled becomes witness to an unmoving center. In Sanskrit, the word for health is *svastha*—*sva* meaning "self," and *stha* meaning "to be situated." From an Ayurvedic perspective, health is to be wholly situated within oneself, bringing consciousness to all of our being, dissolving hard boundaries to enter a world that is inherently balanced, fluid, and free—connecting with the principle of cosmic harmony, and upholding our role or part.

For *Āyurveda*, the concept of balance also exists through paired, complementary forces. In the cosmic realm, *Prakriti*, the divine feminine that manifests material nature, is paired with *Purusha*, the divine masculine, all-encompassing, passive emptiness that is the foundation of all. The unity of these opposites enables life. In everyday existence, the principle of balancing opposites exists in all qualities—hot and cold, oily and dry, heavy and light. For example, depending on our nature, we may need more foods with building qualities—cool, oily, heavy, lubricating; or lightening qualities—hot, dry, light, stimulating. Ultimately, for our own health, and the health of the planet, a balance of complementary forces is required.

Beyond paired harmonizing forces, the central tenet of *Āyurveda* focuses on balancing the body's primary managers, the three complementary forces, *vāta*, *pitta*, and *kapha*. Good health reigns when all three *dosha* function fully and are synchronized with each other. If one *dosha* becomes disturbed, the balance is lost, and the disease process begins. At this point, natural intelligence seeks opposites to restore equilibrium. And with growing awareness of the elements and qualities of our own *dosha* mix, we know when we are askew and we can set about reestablishing order. Of course, no mere mortal dwells continually in balance. We live in physical-social-political environments that don't support health and well-being. We eat, travel, and sleep erratically, talk too much, and take foods and medicines we don't understand. Sometimes we think one thing, say another, and do something else; incongruence that weakens our system. Often our personalities swing from dynamic to passive, hot to cold, outgoing to inner upheaval. We've forgotten what balance feels like, so don't know to what we aspire.

Balance is not a static point, a set condition to be achieved and upheld. It's an ongoing, multifaceted, cumulative phenomenon to be approached one day at a time. For *Āyurveda*, by understanding our unique constitution—both at birth and the present day—and approaching health in broad, layered ways, balance becomes possible. When diet and lifestyle consistently move toward balance, the cells of the body relax, and mental harmony and intuition are supported. And the more we seek equilibrium, the easier it is to return. What does it mean to eat to balance your unique constitution? In a general sense, eating to balance the *dosha* involves choosing foods with qualities that help us reduce what is excessive, or increase what is low within our current constitution.

Most often it's the elements of our birth constitution that become excessive. According to *like attracts like*, we most easily accumulate more of

the elements we already have. Eating to balance the *dosha* is about working out what qualities and elements have become excessive in us, then limiting foods and activities that are high in those attributes, while choosing foods and activities with qualities opposite to those we already have.

Two Ayurvedic Tenets Summarize the Healing Approach

Toward achieving and maintaining *dosha* balance, *Āyurveda* employs two cosmic principles. The first is *like attracts like*, which tells us that *like* qualities attract more of their own, thus increasing in strength, putting us in danger of creating excess. A common cause of *dosha* imbalance is the habitual intake of foods with qualities similar to our own. Consciously or unconsciously, we are drawn to foods and activities with more of the qualities we already have. This occurs more readily when the body is already imbalanced. The second tenet is *opposites reduce*, which sums up *Āyurveda's* rational therapeutic approach. Opposite qualities decrease one another. To restore and support *dosha* balance we should choose foods with qualities opposite to those we have in abundance. At first, we may have to make conscious, deliberate choices. Then, with practice, and as balance is restored, harmonizing choices become more natural and intuitive.

Our ease of staying in balance and ability to tolerate certain foods also varies with time and place. Eating to balance the *dosha* also ideally takes into account our locality and daily cycles and seasons. This may sound complex, but is simply about becoming aware of the elements and qualities dominating in the immediate environment, and understanding how they interact with our own. We look at the practicalities of eating with daily cycles and seasons in Part II on page 109. For now, when it comes to choosing complementary foods, one of the easiest and most enjoyable ways to balance your constitution is to eat for taste. Let's look at the concept of taste, and why for *Āyurveda* the way foods taste is a key aspect of overall health and well-being.

Elevate Taste

Western taste experts consider the human palate able to detect five distinct tastes: sweet, sour, salty, bitter, and umami. While the first four tastes are somewhat intuitive and can be perceived in their pure form, the newest group member, umami, is a little different. Derived from the Japanese word for *delicious*, umami is a meaty flavor, accentuated by protein breakdown during food ripening, cooking, and fermentation. Natural umami flavors occur in vine-ripened tomatoes, shiitake mushrooms, tuna, and processed foods including strong cheeses, cured ham, and cooked food combinations.[3]

Based on our evolutionary past, hungry humans are primed to seek sweetness, signaling a rich source of sugars to fuel the brain and body, and salt, an essential mineral required by every cell. All the while being repelled by bitter and sour flavors associated with bitter plant alkaloids and the acidic rot of decaying food, both potential toxins to the human system. Today, these innate tendencies generate dietary choices that compromise nutrition, but for many Westerners, the concept of taste is pleasure-driven and largely incidental to health. Many snacks and meals are dominated by concentrated artificial flavors that make it impossible to discern and describe subtle tastes. Chefs, good cooks, and fine diners are among the few who understand the skill and importance of balancing flavors to truly please the palate.

From an Ayurvedic perspective, taste is a crucial sensory activity, and six primary tastes exist—sweet, sour, salty, pungent, bitter, and astringent. Importantly, each taste is created through a mix of the five great elements. All elements are contained in all substances, but tastes arise because

---

3   The identification of the umami flavor is credited to the Japanese scientist, Kikunae Ikeda, in 1908. Intrigued by the delicious taste of kombu seaweed broth, Ikeda isolated the source to glutamates; a discovery that somewhat regrettably led to the industrialized manufacture of the flavor enhancer, monosodium glutamate (MSG, or additive 621).

certain elements dominate. Based on the flavor(s) presented, the body recognizes the mix of elements, and primes the digestive fires. The importance and impact of taste also ventures far beyond the tongue. Long after the meal is eaten, the taste of food continues to affect the food body through a *post-digestive taste*, and through the quality of the serum produced that forms the basis of all physical tissues.

The Elements and Qualities Dominating in Each Taste

In each taste two of the five great elements dominates, which introduce their particular qualities and intensities into the body.

Taste	Elements	Qualities
Sweet/ Bland	Earth & Water	cool, moist, heavy, highly building
Sour	Fire & Earth	warm, mildly building
Salty	Fire & Water	warm, moist, mildly building
Pungent	Fire & Air	hot, dry, light, highly reducing
Bitter	Air & Ether	cold, dry, light, highly reducing
Astringent	Earth & Air	cool, hard, heavy, reducing

Taste also affects the mind. Sweet tastes are pleasing and soothing, but in excess can enhance lethargy and desires; sour tastes are refreshing and awakening, but can trigger envy and irritation; salty tastes are grounding and calming, yet can generate impatience and greed; spicy or pungent flavors open the mind and senses, yet can incite anger; bitter tastes are clearing and calming, but can nurture anxiety and grief; and astringent tastes are cooling and contracting, but are aligned with fear and worry. Infinite taste combinations exist, but in most foods, one primary taste is perceived clearly. Secondary tastes are often also present, sometimes recognized at the end of eating.

According to *Āyurveda*, optimal nutrition and balanced *dosha* are contingent on including all six tastes in the daily diet, adjusting the amounts corresponding to personal constitution and cosmic season. Accordingly, certain tastes should be emphasized, and others reduced. Too much or too little of one flavor downgrades its beneficial qualities, and eventually leads to imbalance. Let's sample each taste.

Naturally Sweet Tastes

Āyurveda understands sweet tastes as the dominant combination of earth and water. These elements combine to create sweet tastes with cool, moist, heavy, and building qualities. Historically, thoughts of sweet tastes conjured visions of sun-ripened fruits. Today, fruits taste less sweet, and it is processed junk foods that feed our sweet tooth. But rather than provide cool, moist nourishment, refined concentrated sugars and artificially sweetened foods heat, acidify, and dry the body, impoverish digestion, and leech calcium and other nutrients from the system.

From an Ayurvedic perspective, the sweet taste refers to whole foods that are naturally sweet; foods that tend to stick in the mouth, and provide pleasure and contentment. Sweet foods range in intensity from ripe tropical fruits, sugarcane, jaggery[4], maple syrup, and honey[5]; to cool-weather fruits, squash, fresh dairy foods, seeds, and nuts; to the more bland, neutral flavors of starchy vegetables, whole grain cereals, legumes, meats, and oils. Biochemically, sweet tastes tend to arise from the three macronutrients: carbohydrates, protein, and fat. Across the spectrum, more than three quarters of all whole foods are sweet in taste.

When consumed in balance, the dominant earth and water elements provide naturally sweet and bland-tasting foods with benefits for all *dosha* types. The benefits of sweet foods include:

- Supporting physical growth and building
- Promoting fertility and reproduction; increasing breast milk in lactating women
- Stabilizing and healing wounds, including bone fractures
- Cooling, rejuvenating, and vitalizing the body, mind, and senses
- Stimulating saliva, and relieving thirst
- Promoting pleasure, satisfaction, and love

In particular, the cool, damp, heavy, building qualities of many sweet and neutral tastes help to calm *pitta's* fires, and nourish *vata's* dry, light nature. Those dominant in *kapha dosha*, being already relatively cool, moist, and heavy, should limit sweet tastes. For mixed *pitta-vata* individuals, naturally sweet/bland flavors can be especially helpful.

---

4   *Jaggery* is the primary extraction of sugar cane juice, crystallized into a sweet, highly nutritious, caramelized mass used to flavor Indian sweets and many dishes.
5   While honey offers intense sweetness, it is also astringent and has the special action of heating and drying. This deviation from the rule marks honey as a potent food that, when used correctly, strongly supports healing.

When eaten to excess, naturally sweet-tasting foods result in excess *kapha dosha*, evidenced by congestions such as coughs and colds, obstructions such as clogged arteries (arterio-sclerosis), weak digestion, weight gain, growth of yeasts (Candida) and tumors, laziness, and attachments.

Sour Tastes

In their elemental mix, sour tastes predominate in fire and earth. This blend provides sour foods with a slow-burning heat, some moist- ness and lightness, and mildly building qual-ities. Biochemically, sour tastes derive from plant-based organic acids. Sour foods include grapefruits, limes, and lemons; varieties of apple, grape, and plum; unripe fruits; tomatoes; rosehips; tamarind; vinegar; sauerkraut; olives, and pickled vegetables; aged cheeses and natu-ral yogurts; and foods that are stale and rancid. All fermented foods are sour, including yeasted breads and alcohol, which undergo commercial processes that render them excessively heating and drying and damaging to the digestion.

When consumed in balance and moderation, the dominant fire and earth elements provide naturally sour tastes with benefits for all *dosha* types. The benefits of sour foods include:

- Stimulating and supporting digestion
- Nourishing and strengthening tissues
- Fueling the secretion of bodily fluids
- Helping circulation and elimination
- Relieving thirst, and refreshing the mouth and sense of taste
- Promoting mental determination

> In particular, the heating, building qualities of sour foods nourish and warm *vāta dosha*. In excess, however, sour tastes liquefy and aggravate *kapha*; and can overheat *pitta*. Of the mixed constitutions, *kapha-pitta* individuals should exercise the most restraint and moderation.

In general, too much sour taste acidifies, fer-ments, and degenerates the food body. Excess sour reduces strength and fertility, and promotes flabbiness, premature aging, and issues such as dental sensitivity, hyperacidity, heartburn, ulcers, psoriasis, dermatitis, inflamed eczema, and overly judgmental attitudes.

Salty Tastes

The *Charaka Samhitā* sees salty tastes as mostly composed of the elements fire and water which provide salty foods with mildly warming, sharp, unctuous, heavy qualities. Most salty tastes originate from complex mineral salts. Used on fresh foods and in cooking, salts heighten flavor and sweetness, reduce bitterness, and make food delicious. Examples of salty substances include rock salts, sea salts, refined table salt, and salty compounds such as asafoetida (hing)[6]. More complex, less intense forms include kelp and seaweeds, cheeses, and soy sauce. Today, most dietary salt comes from processed foods.

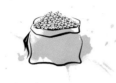

When consumed in balance and moderation, naturally salty foods have the following benefits:

- Increase physical hunger, and promote digestion and assimilation
- Stimulate saliva and secretions; assist stool evacuation, decongestion, and deep cleansing
- Help maintain the body's fluid, mineral, and electrolyte balance
- Promote mental enthusiasm, satisfaction, and grounding

Extreme salty flavors overpower taste, are highly heating, and dry the body. Chronically high intakes of refined salt reliably result in water retention and high blood pressure (hypertension). According to *Āyurveda*, overconsumption of salt causes inflammation, skin disease, gray hair and balding, wrinkles and premature aging, weakness, agitation, and impotence.

> The warm, moist qualities of balanced salty flavors support *vāta dosha*. But the water element aggravates *kapha dosha*. And too much damp heat irritates *pitta* types, who are already high in these qualities. All mixed constitutions, especially *kapha-pitta* types, should limit salty foods and added salts.

Pungent (Spicy) Tastes

Composed chiefly of the elements of fire and air, pungent tastes bring hot, dry, light qualities into the body. Unlike the slow burn of fire and earth (sour tastes), fueled by fire and air, pungent (spicy) tastes burn fast and hot. Pungent heat scalds, but dissipates quickly. Biochemically, spicy tastes emanate from aromatic and acrid plant-based essential oils. Chili and cayenne peppers are highly spicy foods. Less intense pungent foods include black pepper, mustard seeds (and mustard

---

6 Asafetida or *hing* is a pungent resin used in Indian cuisine. A pinch added to cooking water assists thorough cooking and softening of beans and legumes. Many Ayurvedic herbal powders include *hing* as a calming digestive, useful for windy *vāta* types.

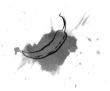

greens), fresh and dried ginger root, and members of the onion family, including scallion and garlic. Spices and herbs of mild pungency include cinnamon, cardamom, clove, fennel, peppermint, spearmint, rosemary, anise, white pepper, horseradish, dill, basil, nutmeg, marjoram, and elderflower. Consumed raw, pungent foods maintain their full force; light steaming preserves most pungency; and longer cooking reduces their burn (such as the difference between raw and cooked garlic).

Consumed in balance and moderation, naturally pungent foods have the following benefits:

- Strongly aid digestion and nutrient absorption
- Remove stagnation; activate the metabolism and cleansing
- Dilate and expand bodily channels, increasing circulation
- Bring out secretions, clearing the eyes, nose, mouth, sinuses, and skin
- Assist with bowel movements, and help to evacuate gas, wastes, parasites, and unhelpful bacteria
- Dry up retained fluid, excess moisture, and fat

- Help to clarify the mind and mentally digest experiences

> The heating, drying, lightening qualities of pungent foods help to balance the cool, moist, heavy qualities of *kapha dosha*. Yet, too much intense heat scorches *pitta*, and the dry, light qualities reliably aggravate *vāta*. Among mixed constitutions, *pitta-vāta* types should tread with extra care.

As with all tastes, balance and moderation are key. Too much pungency in the diet causes excessive thirst, fever and burning, fatigue, fainting, muscle weakness, emaciation, nervous tremors, pain, reduced fertility, and anger.

Bitter Tastes

Composed mostly of air and ether, bitterness brings potent cold, dry, light qualities to the body. Few people consider bitter tastes delicious. Indeed, we are generally repulsed by bitter flavors, associated with bitter plant alkaloids and glycosides (and sour flavors associated with the acidic rot of decaying food), both potential toxins to the human system. Pregnant women become particularly sensitive to bitter tastes to protect the unborn fetus; newborns pucker their lips or poke out their tongue when presented with bitter or sour foods (and smack their lips at the scent of a ripe banana). Yet, in mixed meals, a little bitterness promotes and balances all flavors and provides numerous health benefits. In nature, bitter tastes most often occur in combination with other flavors, as experienced in: celery, lettuce, green leafy vegetables, Brussels sprouts, broccoli, alfalfa, watercress, endive, escarole, dark cabbage leaves, kale, aloe vera, bitter gourd and melon, asparagus, turnip, carrot tops, rhubarb, citrus peel, vinegar, dark chocolate, and coffee. In grains, bitter substances are commonly stored in the germ and husk, experienced in whole grain rye, oats, amaranth, quinoa, and red and black rice. Herbs with bitter notes include echinacea, dandelion root, chicory root, burdock root, yellow dock, turmeric, fenugreek, goldenseal, chamomile, honeysuckle flower, valerian, sandalwood, and chaparral.

When consumed in moderation and balance, bitter foods have the following benefits:

- Strongly lightening and reducing
- Cleanse and purify the blood and all bodily fluids, including breast milk
- Remove undigested toxins (*āma*), and unwanted bacteria and parasites from the gut

- Dry up excess moisture, mucus, fat, and associated damp conditions such as swelling, cysts, tumors, and yeast overgrowth (Candida)
- Relieve excess body heat and fever
- Promote appetite, digestion, liver function, and relieve nausea and intestinal gas
- Cleanse and clear the palate, and restore the sense of taste
- Increase introspection and intelligence

> The strong cooling, drying, lightening qualities of air and ether help to balance overheated or overfed *pitta* types, and damp or overfed *kapha* types, and mixed *pitta-kapha* constitutions. In contrast, strong or excessive bitter flavors reliably aggravate *vāta* types, and should be minimal and mild.

Beneficial as it is, excessive bitterness depletes all bodily tissues, causes coldness, roughness, stiffness, fatigue, emaciation, hair loss, headaches, nervous disorders, and reduces fertility.

Astringent Tastes
Composed chiefly of earth and air, astringent tastes introduce cold, dry, heavy qualities into the body. In nature, astringent tastes rarely dominate, and are least common among the tastes.

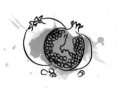

More than a distinct flavor, astringency is experienced as a drying, puckering effect on the tongue, mouth, and throat. Biochemically, the astringent taste stems from plant-based tannins. Astringency is present in unripe bananas, pomegranates, cranberries, many fruit skins, green beans, okra, asparagus, artichoke, garbanzos, yellow split peas, lentils and beans, goldenseal, alfalfa, honey, and black tea. Chlorophyll contains astringency, so all green plants, especially when raw, are slightly astringent.

When consumed in balance and moderation, astringent foods have the following benefits:

- Dry up excess moisture and fat
- Cleanse the blood, sweat, and bowel
- Constrict tissues and channels, and support muscle tissue and tone
- Reduce discharges and unruly bleeding
- Soothe the gut's mucus lining and promote healing
- Assist micronutrient absorption
- Promote mental integrity

The cool heaviness of astringent tastes calm *pitta's* hot, light fires, and the drying, reducing qualities are useful to combat moist *kapha* excess. Being cool, dry, and reducing, too much astringency readily aggravates *vāta*. It is a valuable taste for mixed *pitta-kapha* constitutions.

Overconsumption of astringent foods and fluids brings on a parched tongue or throat, choking feelings, and diminished taste. Channels become dry and constricted, causing poor digestion and circulation, constipation, cramps, bloating, and emotional repression. Emaciation, neuromuscular diseases, nervous disorders, and decreased reproductive fluids and sex drive are other possible consequences.

Pure forms of taste are stronger and potentially more aggravating than mixed, complex flavors. According to *Āyurveda*, a balanced, wholesome diet includes all six tastes, every day, in intensities and proportions that support each unique constitution. For all *dosha* types, sweet/bland-tasting foods should make up the bulk of the diet, plus smaller amounts of naturally sour, salty, pungent, bitter, and astringent foods. We will look at menu plans and approximate proportions in order to put this into practice in Part II on pages 130–133 and 143–152.

Tastes that Balance and Aggravate the *Doshas*

There is an internal logic to choosing foods that provide more of the elements and qualities we lack, and fewer of those we have in abundance. According to your unique constitution, choose foods naturally flavored with balancing tastes, and limit those that are aggravating. In general, people with a dual constitution should focus on balancing, pacifying flavors that overlap both *dosha*. Plus, emphasize tastes that pacify or reduce potentially aggravating qualities during *like* seasons.

Dosha	Balancing, Pacifying Tastes	Aggravating Tastes
Vāta	Sweet/bland; sour; salty	Pungent; bitter; astringent
Pitta	Sweet/ bland; bitter; astringent	Sour; salty; pungent
Kapha	Pungent; bitter; astringent	Sweet/bland; sour; salty
Vāta-Pitta	Sweet/bland	Pungent
Pitta-Kapha	Bitter; astringent	Sour; salty
Vāta-Kapha	*No overlapping tastes*	*No overlapping tastes*

Consider Food's Qualities

The taste attributes of natural foods offer tangible clues about its elemental composition, as well as additional qualities it will bring into the body. Among these qualities, a food's heating or cooling potential is a primary consideration, known to *Āyurveda* as a food's energy or *virya*. Warming foods transfer stimulating, dispersing, lightening properties into the body. Cooling foods calm, contract, and build.

The six tastes offer an immediate indication of the heating or cooling potency of food. Tastes with fire present—pungent, salty, and sour (listed in order of strength)—produce a heating effect. Tastes low in fire—bitter, astringent, and sweet—are immediately cooling in action. Naturally, these heating and cooling effects (and other qualities) differ in strength, and exist along a continuum—greater in pure-tasting foods, and more diffuse in complex foods, and mixed and cooked meals.

Observing the heating and cooling qualities of foods is immensely helpful toward balancing the *dosha*. For warm *pitta* types and those with *pitta* imbalance, balancing tastes—sweet, bitter, and astringent—are low in the fire element, and cooling in nature. For cool *kapha* types and those with *kapha* imbalance, balancing tastes include pungent, bitter, and astringent. The pungent (spicy) taste is the hottest of the flavors and inherently pacifying for *kapha*. The other heating tastes—salty and sour—are less suited due to their moist and building qualities. While bitter and astringent tastes are cooling in nature, their dry, light qualities help pacify *kapha dosha*, and, as we shall shortly see, these two tastes exert further long-term lightening effects on the body. For cold *vāta* types and those with *vāta* imbalance, balancing flavors include the warming tastes of sour and salt, and sweet tastes that, though cooling, are innately moistening and building in nature. The heat of strong pungent tastes is too intense and drying for delicate *vāta*.

The qualities of foods don't readily change, but certain factors can influence their heating or cooling potential. The climate and soil plants are grown in; when and how they are harvested; processing techniques; the part of the plant or animal used; and methods of preparation. Raw foods and foods eaten at room temperature are generally more cooling, while cooking in general, especially long cooking times, dry cooking methods, and high temperatures add heat. Old food and rancid food becomes acidic, and once eaten, also introduces heat. A number of traditional and modern texts catalog the *virya* or thermal potency of foods. These lists can be helpful

to get started, but it's preferable to observe the foods and meals we eat, and the responses within ourselves. The bibliography on page 211 indicates a number of books that list foods and their properties, but due to potential seasonal, geographic, practical, and personal variations, these lists do not always agree.

A food's taste gives an indication of its *immediate* thermal effect—the instant heat of pungent chili, or cool of sweet, bitter, astringent cucumber. *Āyurveda* also recognizes a *post-digestive* taste and effect of food, known as *vipāka*. It takes between six to forty-eight hours for food to move through the gut and liver (depending on what we eat and the rate of digestion). Once digested, the original taste of food often changes and takes on different qualities and distinct long-term actions.

After its initial taste, as the digestive process continues, naturally sweet and salty foods produce a sweet post-digestive essence that exerts a building effect on the body that readily aggravates *kapha dosha* and pacifies *vāta dosha*. After digestion, sour foods remain sour and exert a heating effect that can aggravate *pitta dosha*, and alleviate *vāta* and also *kapha* (if not overdone). Foods that are pungent, bitter, and astringent all become pungent after digestion and exert heating, drying, lightening, reducing effects that are especially helpful for *kapha dosha*, but potentially imbalancing for *vāta* and *pitta*.

The post-digestive effect of sweet and salty foods contributes to the reasons why these tastes disrupt *kapha dosha*, and why it is so hard for many to lose weight. The foods we eat live on in the food body and exert their effects over weeks, months, and years. Those wishing to cleanse the tissues and reduce excess can utilize the qualities of foods and the post-digestive effect by emphasizing pungent, bitter, and astringent tastes, and minimizing those salty and sweet. People wishing to build tissues should reverse this taste emphasis. We examine lightening and building strategies in Chapter 5.

Combine Complementary Qualities
We have a phenomenal variety of foods and foodstuffs at our fingertips. Some foods we eat in their natural form, but mostly we combine foods to make a meal; and most processed foods consist of multiple ingredients. In mixing foods together, we not only combine different ingredients, we combine different qualities as well. Just as certain colors clash and others blend well, so too, depending on their qualities and actions, certain foods work well together, and others conflict and create imbalance.

From an *Āyurveda* perspective, mixing foods and ingredients together can create harmonious tastes and qualities that balance the body, or incompatible tastes and qualities that imbalance the palate and encourage enzyme conflicts, indigestion, *dosha* aggravation, and *āma* (undigested toxins). The ancient sages considered mismatched foods akin to poison. When the qualities and actions of two foods are too dissimilar, or when foods share strong and similar qualities, they are best eaten at separate meals. The following table details some incompatible food combinations.

In general, *Āyurveda* encourages mixed meals that omit foods with contradictory energies, and focuses on complementary food combinations. In everyday terms, poor food combinations include banana milkshakes; fruit *lassis* (churned yogurt, water, and fruit); omelets with cheese or milk; fish or meat with dairy; mixed fruit salads; banana pancakes; a sandwich with a glass of milk; lemon juice on bitter greens; cold liquids with any foods; and hot liquids with other hot or heating foods. Poor food combinations most readily disturb *vāta*-dominant individuals, those with weak digestion, and preexisting *dosha* imbalance. Those with a strong digestion, who are habituated to incompatible foods, or who only take small quantities may experience no

This Food/Food Group:	Is Not Compatible With:
Milk	Bananas; red meats; fish; eggs; beans; yogurt; melons; sour fruits and foods including yeasted breads; green leafy vegetables; garlic
Yogurt	Milk; fish; cheese; starches; beans; sour fruits; melons; mango; banana; dates; all hot drinks and foods
Eggs	Milk; red meats; fish; cheese; fruits; melons; potatoes
Meat	Dairy; honey; sesame seeds
Nightshade vegetables (potatoes, tomatoes, eggplants, peppers)	Yogurt; milk; melon; cucumber
Fruits, especially melons	All foods. (Eat fruits on an empty stomach, or before a meal. Exceptions are lettuce or celery, and grains, which mix with most fruits. Sour fruits—citrus, tomatoes—can be mixed with nuts, seeds, and meats.)
Lemons	Yogurt; milk; cucumber; tomatoes; bitter foods
Grains	Bananas; eggs; milk; dates
Honey	*Ghee* (when taken in equal amounts by weight)
Hot liquids	Meat; fish; dairy including yogurt; other hot foods
Ice cold liquids	All foods (at all times), especially cucumber and melon

ill effects. It's also possible to "antidote" meals high in potentially unbalanced qualities with foods and preparation methods that introduce new qualities to reduce their effects. We explore this practice in Part II on page 135. According to the principles of food combining, the balance of all *doshas* are supported by eating simple meals with fewer ingredients and balanced tastes. For variety, enjoy different food and flavor combinations at each meal.

Eat in an Orderly Fashion

On inspection, the six primary tastes also feature during food digestion. At commencement of the digestive process, in the mouth and top of the stomach, sweet tastes are digested and dominate (stimulating *kapha*). In the bottom of the stomach and throughout the small intestine, sour and salty tastes dominate (stimulating *pitta*). As the process continues, unabsorbed food enters the colon, is dehydrated, and becomes more pungent, bitter, and astringent (stimulating *vāta*). This process by which digesting foods move through six taste stages is reflected in fallen fruits, that move from sweet to fermenting and sour, to pungent, then bitter and astringent decomposition.

Sattva, Rajas, and Tamas
As well as effects on the *dosha* and physical body, *Āyurveda* recognizes that foods contain qualities that affect the mind—and in turn influence the *dosha*. *Āyurveda* speaks of twenty common physical qualities that affect the food body. In addi-

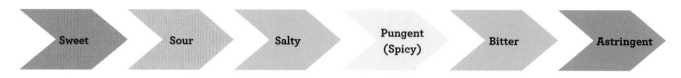

| Sweet | Sour | Salty | Pungent (Spicy) | Bitter | Astringent |

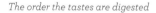
The order the tastes are digested

Given this natural progression, to optimize digestion *Āyurveda* suggests eating foods with dominant tastes in a certain order.

Taste provides flavor, knowledge of a food's major properties and elements, plus it can be used as a guide through which to sequence mixed meals. In practice this means eating naturally sweet foods such as fruits, grains, and sweet vegetables first. According to *Āyurveda*, the beginning of the meal is also the best time to eat dessert! Bitter coffee and astringent teas are best consumed at a meal's end. Without changing any other aspect, modifying the order that you eat certain foods can improve digestive efficiency and support *dosha* balance.

tion, *Āyurveda* and a number of spiritual schools[7] speak of three primary subtle qualities that enter us through foods and exert their effects on the mind. Known as *sattva*, *rajas* and *tamas*, these three complementary forces of Mother Nature are seen to come into existence before the *dosha*, and precede and influence all manifestion.

In the process of creation, *sattva* brings illumination and potential, akin to the dawn of the day. In the psychology, *sattva* supports intelligence, clarity, understanding, intuition, honesty, patience, serenity, flexibility, caring, compassion, non-harming, beauty, joy, humanitarianism, and spiritual consciousness. A mind dominated by *sattva* is present, keenly perceptive, and responds

---

7 Including Vedanta, Samkhya, and Yoga

uniquely to changing contexts. *Sattva* is a passive force, as is *tamas*, while *rajas* is active. *Rajas* is the principle of dynamism; a hot, mobile force, akin to midday, that stimulates mental activity. *Rajas* drives curiosity, expansion, creation, and action, and keeps thoughts and emotions flowing. Too much *rajas* creates instability, hyperactivity, agitation, frustration, impatience, anger, overreaction, aggression, and turbulence. In counterpoint, *tamas* essentially opposes *rajas*. As the principle of substance and inertia, *tamas* offers heaviness, coolness, and restriction; opposing expansion, *tamas* holds mental processes in check. *Tamas* is the dusk of the day, shutting down the senses and delivering us to sleep. When overruled by *tamas*, curiosity and enthusiasm halt. The mind becomes dull, lethargic, and rigid, and stupidity, dishonesty, concealment, repression, delusion, manipulation, greed, and perversion all become possible.

We are all born with a unique combination of the five great elements and three *dosha* that make up our physical nature. But at birth, our essential mental nature is *sattva*—harmonious, peaceful, illuminated, and intelligent. Children are full of *sattva*. They see clearly, learn quickly, and love deeply. From our early days, the mind may already possess some *rajas* and *tamas*, taken on from our mother or father, or carried with us from previous lives. And as life proceeds—through further worldly interactions, the foods we eat, the circumstances and company we keep—we take in more *rajas* and *tamas* and the mind's *sattvic* nature is obscured. In particular, the qualities that govern our early childhood strongly direct the qualities that dominate us as adults.

For the mind to function, *rajas* and *tamas* play a role, but need the support of *sattva*. For example, a *rajasic* mind may animate logic and analysis, but without *sattva's* clarity and intelligence, thought becomes mechanical and heartless (epitomized in modern business and science). A fundamental goal of Vedic and Yogic psychology is to reestablish the elevation of *sattva*. The development of *sattva* cultivates the intelligent principle of discernment and self-observation, and increases the positive attributes of all three *dosha*. To elevate *sattva*, one essential practice is consuming foods high in *sattva*, while avoiding those high in *rajas* and *tamas*. To expand upon these ideas, let's examine a range of food groups, and their dominating qualities, as we move toward *dosha* balance. We return to the specific practice of *sattvic* eating in Part II on page 153.

Food Groups and Whole Foods

When it comes food, *Āyurveda* takes an inclusive view, and recognizes all natural foods as potentially healing; even biological poisons can be medicine in the right dose, at the right time, for the right individual. Many natural foods are mild in their qualities, especially when eaten within dietary variety. Other foods are stronger in nature, concentrated in elements that exert strong effects on the body. When we eat foods high in qualities we already possess, habitual intake naturally leads to *dosha* imbalance. When the foods we choose possess qualities opposing our current imbalance, or complementing our natal constitution, they pacify the *dosha* and promote balance.

For *Āyurveda*, it's not about choosing from or omitting entire food groups or specific foods. Rather than dwell upon *plant-based* or *animal-based*, Ayurvedic wisdom was crafted in times when people related to *whole* plants and *whole* animals within a life philosophy that included the entire ecosystem. Whole foods, wild-crafted by Mother Nature, or raised in or on fertile fields, processed gently and minimally were the foundation of healthy balanced eating. Humans have always eaten both plants and animals, and food production requires both. Plants grow best in the company of animals,

and animals only thrive in association with healthy plants. Untold generations of farmers have known this. Only recently in India and other nations, fraught farmers' relationship with nature has moved from biodiverse and inclusive, to exclusive profit-sighted strategies that kill soils and associated life.

History clearly tells us that not all social change is advantageous. Civilizations that adopt unsustainable practices don't survive.[4] In food production, the division of plants and animals to separate mass production supports deforestation; loss of biodiversity; degradation and poisoning of soil, water, and air; ecological imbalance at local and global levels; animal cruelty; and demise of human life. Mechanization and new technologies render us less able to see ourselves as part of the cycle of soil, water, sun, and life. Yet, only by thinking and living in terms of inclusion rather than exclusion, and wholeness rather than parts, can we truly find personal and global balance.

Over time, a range of Ayurvedic texts have recognized and recorded the qualities of many plants and animals—as heating or cooling, moistening or drying, heavy or light, and high in *sattva*, *rajas*, or *tamas*. The following section addresses various food groups and considers the main qualities of common foods and their relationship with *dosha*. While focusing on theory, this section also contains some practical advice within the context of specific foods. At times, Western food-related concepts and research are raised, including consideration of modern farming and environmental issues.

Vegetables

Most vegetables are comprised of the elements of earth and water, plus various smaller amounts of fire, air, and ether to form a complex range of tastes and qualities. Root vegetables and squash are earthier, sweeter, and denser, tonic, and building. Leafy vegetables such as broccoli, cabbage, kale, and cauliflower tend to be airier, and more bitter and cleansing, with a pungent, reducing *vipāka*. Allium vegetables such as onions, garlic, leeks, chives, scallions, and shallots contain relatively more fire, and are pungent and heating, with a pungent *vipāka*, and introduce *rajas* to the mind. The nightshade vegetables (of the Solanaceae family), including potatoes, tomatoes, eggplants, and peppers, tend also to harbor *rajas*, and contain compounds that can weaken digestion, and aggravate food sensitivities and arthritis, especially in *vāta*, and also in *pitta* types. If sensitive, remove skins and seeds and cook well, or avoid. These foods aside, most vegetables are *sattvic* in nature; their actions balanced and mild.

Rather than rigidly choose vegetables according to *dosha*, they are best chosen according to season and grown fresh and local. Wherever possible, choose organically produced varieties. Seek out heirloom vegetables that are not hybridized or engineered and remain the way nature intended. Grow your own vegetables, and take the time to carefully prepare them. Vegetables are most nutritious when lightly cooked. Eaten raw they are more cooling and reducing—best for *pitta* and robust *kapha* types, in conjunction with a cooked meal. Vegetables combine well with all food groups except fruit.

Fruits

Fruits are perhaps Mother Nature's finest gift—mostly comprised of water and ether, fruits are sweet and complex in taste, packed with nutrients, light to digest, and easily fermented to alcohol. When naturally ripened and chemical free, fruits are cooling, moistening, lightening, cleansing, and supremely *sattvic*, with mild post-digestive actions. When unseasonal, unripe, and grown with chemicals, the beneficial qualities of fruits can be largely negated. Characteristics of wholesome fruit include being seasonal, grown in fertile soils, and having good aroma, color, taste, juice, size, and potency. Ripe fruits contain more enzymes to enhance their digestion. For further enhancement, consume some of all parts of the fruit.

In moderate amounts, ripe seasonal fruits are mild and beneficial for all constitutions—cooling for *pitta* types, hydrating and easy-to-digest for *vāta* individuals, and light and cleansing for those with *kapha* dominance. The coolest part of fruit is the juice, while rinds, skins, pulps, and seeds are relatively warmer, with a pungent *vipāka*. To temper their overall cooling, lightening qualities, *vāta* types can cook fruits with warming spices such as clove, cinnamon, nutmeg, or ginger. Some fruits such as mango, avocado, and banana are naturally nutritive and heavy, and can congest *kapha* types. Especially avocadoes and bananas, with their sweet and sour *vipāka* respectively. Sour fruits are better eaten in the morning, and sweet fruits in the afternoon. Dried fruits are less moist and congesting, and combine well with cereals and grains. In general, however, fruit should be eaten alone or before other foods. Fruits consumed during or on top of a meal stall digestion and encourage fermentation. Wherever possible, choose organic fruits in season. Avoid eating imported, unseasonal fruits daily.

Whole Grains and Cereals

Early man ate grains, but locally-grown, seasonally, and not too many. At the end of a hot, dry summer, sun-bleached grasses gifted seeds—the collection and processing of which required planning and hard work. After hand-gathering and husking, garnered grains were moistened and fermented or sprouted, then ground up, and cooked in water or over flames. In contrast to fruits that can be plucked and eaten, grains require processing and partial digestion before they can be incorporated into the body. Today, at least ten thousand years of cultivation have made grains a mainstay ingredient. Most established cuisines favor one or more loved grains—rice, wheat, barley, rye, corn, buckwheat, sorghum, and millet.

From an Ayurvedic perspective, whole grains are the seed of the plant, its essence of nutrition. Mostly comprised of the earth element, whole grains build tissues, provide stamina, satisfy hunger and taste, and are generally *sattvic*—calming and grounding in nature. The fibrous inner husk removes excess bile and acidity, cleanses the gut, and gives bulk to stool. Most grains are sweet in taste, becoming sweeter when well-cooked and well-chewed, with a sweet, building post-digestive action. Fairly neutral in their qualities, and gentle in action, in general, whole grains balance all constitutions. Brown rice is good for everybody. Wheat is particularly sweet, moist, and heavy, and good for *pitta* and *vāta* types (so long as they can digest it). Oats are mild, grounding, and benefit these types too. Barley is sweet, but lighter and drying, so a good choice for *kapha*. The slight bitterness and astringency of corn, rye, buckwheat, and millet support moist, heavy *kapha*, as does a light dry-roasting before cooking, which renders grains lighter and more warming. Whole grains combine well with each other, and with vegetables, and most other foods. When well stored, they hold their potency, and can be enjoyed in all climates by all constitutions. Avoid all GM grains, and animals that have fed on them.

It's no secret to *Āyurveda* that whole grains inadequately processed, eaten to excess, or consumed as refined products, imbalance digestion and the *dosha*. Not just poorly prepared whole gains, but in particular, refined flours provide no complex nutrients, little bulk, and form a gluey mass that adheres to gut walls and becomes toxic and deeply *tamasic*. This nutritionally depleted, denatured, tacky sludge, blocks channels, hinders digestion, and creates a lush breeding-ground for harmful bacteria. Refined flours—white breads, noodles, pastas, crackers, pastries, and the like—promote gut blockage and inflammation, and dull the mind.

Lectins Revealed

Western science understands whole grains as complex in nutrients, low in fat, and high in dietary fiber with the ability to satisfy hunger. In this way, whole grains, beans, and lentils recently came to the Western table, and looked wholly attractive, until the idea of *lectins* emerged. In plants, lectins organize themselves within the seed husks of beans, peas, and nuts, and the skins and seeds of some fruits and vegetables (particularly the nightshades). Nibbled by rodents or insects, lectins prove mildly toxic, and aim to deter further activity. When seeds are swallowed by humans, they prefer to pass intact out the other end; we cannot digest the hard husks of seeds and grains. But when chewed, these mild plant-based poisons enter the system, and can irritate the gut. Those sensitive to lectins can develop conditions including gut inflammation, bloating, gas, intestinal permeability (leaky gut), allergic responses, arthritis, mental fog, migraines, and weight gain.[5] People high in *vāta dosha* are most at risk. To unlock grains' precious cache, previous generations of cooks understood processes such as storing (one-year-old grains are more digestible than those freshly harvested), soaking, sprouting, acidifying or alkalizing, toasting, grinding, mixing with digestive spices and compounds, long simmering, and most recently, pressure-cooking. Today, such care and knowhow are often missing; alongside food processing and cooking practices that fail to break down these plant-based compounds, and render them more difficult to digest. Further, in selecting for agricultural traits, and probably also in genetic engineering, we have bred less digestible foods. And simultaneously suffer from weak digestion, and a sea of digestive complaints.

As refined flours and sugars enter the blood-stream, they fatigue the pancreas, upset the hormones, heat and acidify the system, and the list goes on. So too, all speed-risen breads (white and whole meal) dry *vāta dosha* through excess air, and provoke *pitta dosha* through the sour heat of fermentation, and all *dosha* through rapidly released sugars. Unleavened whole grain breads such as chapattis/rotis, tortillas, and matzoh are better options.

Those whose family have been preparing and eating whole grains for generations are most likely to be best adapted. After eating whole grains, if you feel affected, focus on how the meal is prepared and consumed. Meal plans in Chapter 9 on page 143 offer further serving advice, and the appendix on page 201 offers details on how to preprocess, cook, and serve whole grains in ways that support meal enjoyment and *dosha* balance. If you suspect you are intolerant of a grain (often wheat), see Chapter 8 on page 120 for advice on how to identify problem foods. Often, as grain choice, quantity, and preparation methods improve, and the body heals, whole grains and other complex foods are better tolerated and enjoyed.

Beans, Lentils, and Peas

Many traditional cuisines incorporate legumes, but perhaps none more than the varied dishes of the Indian subcontinent. Every menu features beans (aduki, fava, kidney, flat, lima, soy), lentils (red, black, green, whole, split), peas (green, garbanzo/chickpea), and sometimes peanuts, mixed with tasty, digestive spices. Legumes are comprised mostly of the elements of earth and air. Sweet and astringent in taste, cooling, with a sweet *vipāka*, they nourish and strengthen, but can also be rough, drying, gas-forming, heavy, and hard to digest. We think of beans and lentils as promoting bowel function, but in excess or improperly prepared they upset digestion and cause constipation. With air in their mix, legumes are naturally *vāta*-provoking, especially when dried or canned; fresh beans less so; and sweet, moist green beans are harmonizing. To optimize digestion, dried legumes should be presoaked or sprouted, taken in small quantity, and prepared with pungent spices, salts, and fats. The appendix on page 201 offers further advice.

When correctly prepared, those with *pitta* and *kapha* constitution can enjoy legumes regularly—but begin slowly, and don't overdo it. Split mung dal (a small yellow lentil) is easiest to digest, and most suited to *vāta dosha*. The mung bean is the only *sattvic* bean; most beans and lentils introduce *rajas*, and stimulate the mind. Once dried, beans and lentils hold their properties, and can be eaten year-round, though may be best-digested in winter. Legumes combine well with sweet, earthy vegetables, and grains, such as the marriage of lentils and rice in *kitchari* (see recipe on page 202). In *dal* (thick lentil curry), a range of lentil varieties can be used, and may be mixed in the same dish. As a crop, legumes are particularly benevolent. They absorb a significant amount of atmospheric nitrogen, and provide nutrients to the soil.

Nuts, Seeds, and Oils

Nuts and seeds are generally dominated by earth and fire. Sweet, warming, and heavy, with a sweet, building post-digestive action, *Āyurveda* considers them one of the most potent foods available—encapsulating the reproductive potential of plants and trees: almonds, cashews, hazelnuts, walnuts, macadamia, pecan, brazil, pistachio, coconut, pine nuts, and sesame, pumpkin, sunflower, flax, and chia seeds. Freshly-shelled seeds and nuts nourish all tissues, and are innately *sattvic* and rejuvenating. However, once removed from their husk or shell, oils oxidize rapidly. Rather than benefit the body, rancid nuts, seeds, and oils create inflammatory effects. The oils of nuts and seeds are also highly susceptible to accumulate oil-based agrochemicals. To enjoy the benefits of nuts and seeds, prioritize fresh, organic produce.

The dense nourishing oiliness of nuts and seeds suits light, dry *vāta* types best (when freshly prepared, well-chewed, and eaten in moderation), and least benefits heavy, moist *kapha*. Small amounts of pumpkin, flax, and chia seeds, and unsalted pistachios are generally best tolerated by those with damp *kapha* conditions. In summer, the warming quality of nuts and seeds can aggravate *pitta*; they are best taken in winter and fall. According to *Āyurveda*, a serving of nuts is three (three!) per day. Two per day if the individual is small or with weak digestion. To improve digestibility (especially for *vāta* types), soak seeds and nuts overnight to dilute and activate them. Then, removing the outer skins before eating expels most anti-nutrients. A light dry-roasting is also useful to reduce heaviness, and any effects of rancidity—but too much heat denatures sensitive oils, and makes them heavy and hard to digest. Freshly ground nut butters; raw, cold-pressed oils; and fresh or fermented nut milks are other ways to benefit from seeds and nuts, especially if chewing or digestion are weak. Wherever possible opt for organic. Avoid pre-chopped nuts, slivered almonds, and cheap nut butters that contain the poorest quality ingredients.

Nuts and seeds can be eaten alone, or combined with most fruits, grains, and non-starchy vegetables. Purchase small quantities, preferably in-shell, or sealed in vacuum-packing. Store your produce in airtight glass, away from heat and light.

The Juice on Fats

From an Ayurvedic perspective, dietary fats are an essential part of healthy eating; the question is of quality and balance. For the food body, fats are mostly sweet, rejuvenating, and energizing, with a sweet, building *vipāka*. Fatty substances render cell walls firm yet flexible, and moisten and support all tissues. Oils are a chief component in all lubricating tissues including cerebrospinal fluid and synovial fluid in joints. During digestion, oils lubricate, insulate, and nourish *pitta's* fires. Throughout the physical body fats protect vital organs and insulate against excess heat and cold. In accidents and times of shock, fats shield us and help guard against loss of physical structure. From an Ayurvedic perspective, oils are a chief component in all bodily fluids and, essential in the body's fluid metabolism. In general, fats provide strength and energy; aid rejuvenation; offer grounding, contentment, and security; and enable supple, lustrous skin, and glossy hair.

Among humans and other animals, high fat foods are innately preferred. Our hunter ancestors selectively sought well-padded terrestrial herbivores and oily sea-faring creatures. Successful huntsmen were given first pick of the life-sustaining delicacies of brains, livers, tails, and fatty depots cushioning the eyeballs and kidneys. On the palate, fats carry taste and enhance rich flavors. In the mouth, fats provide a creamy coating on the cheeks and tongue. To the nose, fried fats create succulent aromas. To the ears, fats sizzle. To the eyes, fats glisten. And in the stomach, fatty foods satisfy.

We all benefit from dietary fats, but those who benefit most are thin, dry, or nervous. In general, *vāta* types need greater amounts of oils (so long as they can digest them), *pitta* types require moderate to low amounts, and *kapha* types need little and least. Part II on page 143 provides guidance on specific *dosha*-appropriate fats and oils, but in general, *Āyurveda's* favorite plant-based oils come from sesame and coconut. Both oils have long been used in many Eastern cultures. Sesame oil is sweet, bitter, pungent, and astringent, immediately warming with a sweet, building *vipāka*, and is subtle (can penetrate fine channels), and digestible. Coconut oil is sweet and cooling, with a sweet, building vipāka. It is heavy, yet digestible in moderation. Both oils are highly nutritious, enhance beauty and intelligence, and are relatively shelf- and cooking-stable, and easily cold-pressed. Sesame oil is favored for external massage and cleansing therapies, while coconut oil is more cooling and soothing. Overuse of either oil readily congests *kapha* types.

In general, keep the following points in mind when choosing and using dietary oils and fats:

- *Avoid refined oils.* That an oil is *refined* may sound pleasing, but it means the oil has been extracted using chemical and caustic solvents and/or temperatures as high as 600°F (316°C), then bleached to a desirable color, and deodorized through more high-temperature processing.
- *Avoid hydrogenated oils.* Hydrogenation produces unnatural *trans* fats; destroys essential fatty acids, fat-soluble vitamins, antioxidants, and untold other constituents; introduces *free radicals* that only survive for a nanosecond, yet trigger chain reactions that inflame, stress, and age cell walls and membranes; and ravage our lipid metabolism.
- *Avoid deep-fried foods and commercial meals and snacks containing refined oils.* Most pastries, biscuits, cakes, snack foods, frozen dinners, pastes, and sauces are invariably made with refined and hydrogenated oils. Removing these substances from the diet is key in healing *kapha* accumulation, alleviating inflammation and excess *pitta*, and supporting *vāta's* delicate nerves and tissues.
- *Choose chemical-free, cold-pressed oils.* Unless an oil is clearly labelled "cold-pressed," chances are it has been extracted using chemicals and/or heat.
- *Choose oils labelled extra virgin* or *unrefined.* These oils contain integral plant constituents needed to fully digest the oil and nourish the body.
- *Choose freshly extracted oils.* Check the date of manufacture, and purchase and use within six months. Store all oils in tightly sealed, darkened glass containers in a cool, dark place to protect this sensitive nectar from air, light, and heat.
- *Favor monounsaturated fats (that are chemical-free, cold-pressed, and fresh).* Oils with this fatty acid arrangement are more shelf-stable, and stable in cooking. Monounsaturated fatty acids are high in oils made from olives, avocados, almonds, apricot kernels, peanuts (ground nuts), canola, and "high oleic" sunflower seeds. Sesame oil contains less than fifty percent monounsaturated fats, but comprises nearly equal quantities of polyunsaturated fats, an

arrangement which supports shelf life and cooking stability.

- *When cooking, don't overheat oils.* Use low heat, and heavy bottomed pans. Start with a little water in the pan before adding oil. This reduces the heat the oil is exposed to, and supports less use of oil.
- *Oils are ideally enjoyed unheated.* Rather than frying foods, after cooking, add a drizzle of oil over warm vegetable and grain dishes and salads.
- In addition to extracted oils, use fresh whole foods such as nuts and seeds.

Naturally, the food body manufactures oils and fats closely resembling the composition of those we consume. When poor in quality, high-fat diets promote hard-to-shift weight gain, gallbladder and liver dysfunction, heart disease, diabetes, tumors and cancers, and many other modern-day degenerative and chronic conditions.

Meat and Animal Products

A flick through the *Charaka Samhitā* and *Madanapāla's Nighantu*, a fourteenth century *materia medica* of *Āyurveda*, informs the dominant qualities of animals including bear, lion, crocodile, donkey, dog, jackal, fish, mouse, and vulture, and different types of honey, milk products, skin, blood, flesh, fats, bone, marrow, semen, bile, feces, urine, horn, nail, hoof, and hair. In general, animals are classified based on how and what they eat, and the environment they inhabit. Flesh from different parts of the animal also possesses different qualities. Overall, animal flesh is dominant in the earth element, plus water and fire. Animal flesh is sweet, salty, sour, and pungent in taste; warming; sweet and building in post-digestive action; and heavier in nature than vegetables, legumes, and grains. Good quality meat is freshly killed, from a strong animal that is not diseased, contaminated, or emaciated, and did not die of drowning or poisoning. All other meat harbors *rajas* and *tamas*, aggravates all *doshas*, readily creates *āma*, and should be avoided.

In general, wild game from desert regions is considered lightest, least heating, less oily, and more readily digestible than other meats, and the only flesh suitable for regular consumption. Goat, chicken, and turkey are also relatively light; while beef, pork, lamb, and fish are generally exceedingly heating (aggravate *pitta*), congesting (aggravate *kapha*), and heavy to digest (aggravate *vāta* and sensitive or slow digestions). Traditionally, *vāta* types and individuals who are weak, emaciated, or convalescing were given broths and soups made from robust, freshly killed animals. From soups, even without eating meat, nutrients can be readily extracted.

So long as *vāta* types can digest it, in moderation, the warming, heavy, building qualities of meat can support *dosha* balance. *Pitta* types generally have a strong digestion, but the warm, moist, acidic qualities of flesh aggravate their fire and water elements which are already high. For *kapha* types, the slow, dense heaviness of meat is a digestive challenge, and its oily, heavy qualities congest and naturally build tissues. Pure *pitta* and *kapha* constitutions do best by limiting meat consumption, and often do well as vegetarians.

Historically, the types of meat people ate and how much was less often a health consideration, and more often related to availability and sometimes religion. The East African Maasai and Arctic Inuit have traditionally dined almost exclusively on animals and their products, supporting robust humans and successful societies. Most traditional accounts of killing or hunting emphasize the act as a moment of deep reverence and compassion; of gratitude to the animal that gives its life. In the Hindu caste system, the Brahmins or priestly caste were mainly vegetarian. The ruling classes, however, lauded hunting and meaty banquets. The warrior caste ate meat for its heaviness and stamina, and perhaps to support a bloodthirsty mindset. Wealthy landowners farmed large beasts. Businessmen acclaimed meat for its taste and symbol of prosperity and

status. Lower classes kept household pigs and chickens, and enjoyed meat for its warmth, nourishment, and heaviness in the belly. Dairy and eggs were common to all classes. The sacred cow, however, was never harmed or eaten—an observance with practical and spiritual roots. In other spiritual circles, Buddhists, Tantrics, and Taoists traditionally avoid meat. The great twentieth-century Indian saint, Ramana Maharishi, advocated the avoidance of meat as a key practice to open and clarify the mind, and move closer to one's essential nature.

Today, other reasons why people choose not to eat meat include ethical issues related to animal cruelty; issues of environmental sustainability linked with methods of contemporary commercial production; and for reasons of health related to concerns about safety, toxins, and links between high meat consumption and cancers and other diseases. Eating high on the food chain exposes us to a phenomenon called *bio-concentration*. Commercial farming douses plants with chemicals that accumulate in the oily parts of grains that are then fed to cows, pigs, chicken, and fish. Through the course of their life, these animals assimilate herbicides, pesticides, fungicides, heavy metals, antibiotics, recombinant hormones, *āma*, and other poisons in their tissues at concentrations thousands of times their original levels. When these animals become human food, the body takes this on.

Commercially farmed livestock are housed in toxic environments, and fish—free-living and farmed—suffer a similar fate. Most salt and freshwater fish grow in polluted waters and accumulate biohazards such as methylmercury, poly-carbonated biphenyls (PCBs), dioxins, and plastic residues. Rampant overfishing has pushed marine environments and fish populations to the brink, while farmed fish are intensely raised in polluted waters and fed chemicals and often genetically engineered grains. Despite these unfortunate circumstances, fish (especially varieties of mackerel, trout, herring, sardines, albacore tuna, salmon, and halibut) serve as primary sources of long-chain, polyunsaturated, omega-3 fatty acids. Fish and other meat and animal products are also held in high stead as good sources of *protein*.

By association, animal products such as dairy foods and eggs contain many similar qualities to the animals they come from. Eggs are warming, moist, and heavy, with a sweet, building *vipāka*, but can be easier to digest than meat, and are useful for *vāta* types, and in healing. Of all animal products, *Āyurveda's* favorite is definitely unctuous, nourishing, *sattvic* milk from happy,

Pushing Protein

Since the three macronutrients—carbohydrates, fat, and protein—were discovered a couple of hundred years ago, the concept of high-protein foods and their dietary imperative has rung in medical thinking and in today's collective psyche. Indeed, the word protein derives from the Greek word *proteios*, meaning "primary substance" or "holding first place." The food industry asks: *have you had your protein today?* And industry influences have inclined Western dietary guidelines toward recommending multiple daily servings of protein-rich foods[6]. In mainstream circles, "high-protein" foods have become synonymous with a wholesome diet. Plus, based on limited and changeable criteria, we have been programmed to think of animal-based protein as *high quality* and plant-based protein as *inferior*. While historically, entire civilizations, including the ancient Indians, Egyptians, Mexicans, and Chinese, obtained the bulk of dietary protein from relatively low-protein foods including whole wheat, rice, and corn, *Āyurveda* does not think in terms of single nutrients, instead understanding that all substances function within living complexes, and that too little or too much of any one constituent will inevitably imbalance the *dosha* and initiate disease.

grass-fed cows. Rather than heating, cow's milk is a sweet, cooling substance that is sweet and building in post-digestive action, healing, rejuvenating, and promoting of *ojas* and intelligence. Freshly boiled and warm with raw sugar and digestive spices, milk is calming for *vāta*. Fresh and room temperature, milk is cooling for *pitta*. Yet the cool, heavy building qualities of milk (and most dairy products) are mucus-promoting and aggravating for *kapha dosha*.

Traditionally in Indian culture, fresh milk was boiled, and an acid (yogurt or lemon juice) was added to curdle the milk to create a fresh cheese known as *paneer*, which is lightly fried and added to curries, often together with puréed spinach. All cheeses tend to be heavy, building, and congesting, with a sour post-digestive action, but fresh cheeses such as *paneer* and cottage cheese are cooler and lighter to digest. Fermented and salted cheeses are more warming and heavy. Fresh milk was also often fermented to yogurt, an unctuous, warming, building food with a sour, building *vipāka*, that in small quantities aids appetite and digestion. As it is heavy and congesting, yogurt is best churned with water to create *lassi* (in a ratio of 1:1 to 1:4). See the appendix on page 206 for *lassi* recipes to suit all constitutions. All dairy is most suited to *vāta* types, and is best avoided at night and during spring, and in *kapha* aggravation.

Golden *Ghee*

Traditionally, *ghee* was made from the milk of grazing animals, most often from cows, prepared from milk fermented into yogurt, then churned to butter, before being gently simmered to separate and remove the solid fraction. The remaining golden liquid is a sweet, unctuous oil that is subtle enough to take on the qualities of the substances it is mixed with, and enter deep tissues. In its processing, *ghee* is predigested three times. First by the cow in the making of milk; second while churned to butter, and third while the butter is heated to produce *ghee*. Add a fourth digestion if the milk is fermented to yogurt, but nowadays unsalted butter is used. Upon consumption, golden *ghee* kindles the digestive fires, enhances *ojas*, and nourishes and cleanses the system, including the eyes, reproductive functions, and mind, and promotes tissue gain in convalescing individuals. The sweet, cooling qualities of *ghee*, and its sweet post-digestive actions, hydrate and pacify heat, inflammation, and acidity—good to soothe *pitta*, so long as it's not too building (bitter "*tikta*" *ghee* can be particularly useful). For *vāta dosha*, *ghee's* unctuous, building qualities readily soften and pacify. In *kapha* types, *ghee's* sweet, cold, oily qualities are aggravating, but can be alleviating in small amounts paired with pungent substances. In the kitchen *ghee* is shelf-stable against oxidation; in cooking it does not break down, or burn easily like butter; and in meals it adds gloss and promotes rich, sweet, nutty flavors.

In Indian culture yogurt was also further processed to make butter, buttermilk, and eventually *ghee*. Butter is considered sweet, cooling, unctuous, heavy, and congesting and difficult to digest. Buttermilk, the liquid remaining after butter production, is slightly warming, lighter, and less mucus forming, and an easy food to digest (commercial varieties less so). And *ghee*, or clarified butter, is cooling, moistening, heavy, and building, yet stimulates and balances the digestive fires, and is considered *sattvic*, nourishing, and rejuvenating second to none.

Today we are far removed from the cows that give us their daily milk and dairy. By Ayurvedic standards, highly processed commercial milks are classed as poison—an amalgam from chemically treated, factory raised cows, that is subsequently separated, reconstituted, homogenized, and pasteurized. The modern-day obsession with separating components, altering fat levels, and super-heating to kill bacteria renders milk largely indigestible. Yet, milk often maintains lifelong emotional significance—the milk of the mother still casts its spell, while many milk and dairy devotees would do much better without. Milk is one of the most common self-reported food allergens in the world.[7] Instead of an elixir, consumption of commercial cow's milk has been linked with increased risk of sinus allergies and Candida, some cancers, osteoporosis and bone fractures[8], and multiple sclerosis.[9] And infants weaned on to cow's milk have a higher risk of type-1 diabetes.[10]

While animal products were common on most traditional menus, they featured more as a supplementary bonus than daily norm. Most societies did not eat meat every day—let alone at multiple meals. From an Ayurvedic perspective, all constitutions should consider portions of meat and animal products more as condiments than the centerpiece of a meal. As well as supporting digestability, *Āyurveda* and yoga recognize that flesh introduces *rajas* to the mind that unsettles and promotes hyperactivity; as well as the heavy, sluggish, dull qualities of *tamas*. Together, both *rajas* and *tamas* feed aggression and primal yearnings that anchor us in material turmoil. Further, animals raised, milked, and killed in fear and violence are bound to store these emotions into their tissues, and transmit them to the eater. Always choose fresh meats, milks, and animals products derived from animals naturally and ethically raised without hormones or chemicals.

Herbs and Spices

Herbs and spices are concentrated foods, and an integral part of Ayurvedic strategies to enliven and balance meals, support digestion, cleanse the system, and balance the *dosha*. In practical use, choose varieties that are fresh, chemical-free, and locally grown. Plants cultivated in soils, waters, air, and climatic conditions local to ourselves are more aligned with the food body, adapted to support life in that area. Grow herbs at home. Select herbs and spices for their tastes, aromas, qualities, actions, colors, textures, and according to intuition. Borrow ideas from different cultural cuisines. Lightly toast whole spices to bring out their flavor, aroma, and digestive potential.

Grind dry whole seeds and spices as you need them in a mortar and pestle, or pulse in a coffee grinder. Add fresh herbs at the end of cooking or sprinkle over a warm meal. Do the same with fresh ginger. Make fresh herb chutneys. After eating, chew a pinch of dry roasted spices such as fennel or cumin, or steep for tea. Experiment with all six tastes.

The following table lists the qualities, *dosha* effects, and benefits of common Indian and Western spices.

Common Name *Botanical Name*	Qualities [vipāka] Effect on *Dosha* (V, P, K) "-" reduce/pacify; "+" increase/ aggravate; "=" neutral effect	Benefits
Ajwain (Carom) *Trachyspermum ammi*	Pungent, bitter; hot; sharp; light [pungent—reducing] -KV +P	Digestive; reduces acidity and stomach pain; burns toxins; supports spleen and kidneys; anti-parasitic
Asafoetida (*Hing*) *Ferula assafoetida*	Pungent; hot; *rajasic* [pungent—reducing] -VK +P	Digestive; antispasmodic; burns toxins; decongestive; antiseptic; expels parasites; aphrodisiac
Basil *Ocimum basilicum*	Sweet, pungent, astringent; hot; *sattvic* [pungent—reducing] -KV +P (in excess)	Digestive; antispasmodic; burns toxins; immune stimulant; decongestant; anti-bacterial; calms the nerves
Bay leaves *Laurus nobilis*	Sweet, pungent, astringent; hot [pungent—reducing] -KV +P (in excess)	Digestive; assist absorption; reduce acidity; anti-microbial; anti-fungal

Common Name *Botanical Name*	Qualities [vipāka] Effect on *Dosha* (V, P, K) "-" reduce/pacify; "+" increase/ aggravate; "=" neutral effect	Benefits
Black Pepper *Piper nigrum*	Pungent; hot; light; dry; *rajasic* [pungent—reducing] -KV +P	Digestive; burns mucus and toxins; expels gas, worms, and parasites; blood tonic
Cardamom *Elletaria cardamomum*	Pungent, sweet ; warm, light, dry; *sattvic* [pungent—reducing] -VK =P	Digestive; assists absorption; reduces mucus; burns toxins; antispasmodic; relaxant; heart and mind stimulant
Chili/Cayenne *Capsicum frutescens*	Pungent; hot; sharp, light; *rajasic* [pungent—reducing] -KV +P	Digestive; burns toxins; decongestant; enhances sweating, circulation; expels worms/parasites; aphrodisiac
Cilantro; Coriander *Coriandrum sativum*	Astringent, sweet; cool; *sattvic* [sweet—building] =PKV	Digestive; calming; cleansing; anti- inflammatory; antihistamine; diuretic
Cinnamon *Cinnamomum verum*	Sweet, pungent, astringent; hot; light; *sattvic* [pungent—reducing] -VK +P (in excess)	Assists absorption, assimilation, circulation, cleansing; decongestant; antimicrobial; pain relief; aphrodisiac
Clove *Syzyguim aromaticum*	Pungent, sweet; hot; sharp; oily; *rajasic* [pungent—reducing] -VK +P	Digestive; relieves gas and pain; stimulates sweating; decongestant; anti-microbial; aphrodisiac
Cumin (white) *Cumimum cyminum*	Pungent, bitter; warm; dry; light; *sattvic* [pungent—reducing] -K =VP	Digestive; helps absorption; relieves gas; antispasmodic; diuretic; decongestant; good for blood circulation; anti-microbial
Dill *Anethum graveolens*	Pungent, sweet, astringent; hot; dry; *rajasic* [pungent—reducing] -VK +P (in excess)	Digestive; antispasmodic; relieves gas; expectorant; diuretic; stimulates sweating; anti-microbial
Fennel *Foeniculum vulgare*	Sweet, pungent; warm; light; *sattvic* [sweet—building] =VPK	Stimulates appetite; digestive; antispasmodic; relieves gas and reflux; diuretic

Common Name *Botanical Name*	Qualities [vipāka] Effect on *Dosha* (V, P, K) "-" reduce/pacify; "+" increase/ aggravate; "=" neutral effect	Benefits
Fenugreek *Trigonella foenum-graecum*	Bitter, pungent; hot; sharp; *rajasic/ sattvic* [pungent—reducing] -VK +P	Digestive; decreases acid reflux; soothes membranes; anti-inflammatory; cleanses blood; aphrodisiac; promotes breast milk production
Ginger[8] *Zingiber officinale*	Pungent, sweet; hot; light; oily; *sattvic* (fresh) [sweet—building] -KV +P (in excess)	Digestive; cleansing; antispasmodic; decongestant; anti-inflammatory; anti- nausea; pain relieving
Mustard Seed *Brassica juncea*	Pungent; hot; sharp; oily; *rajasic* [pungent—reducing] -VK +P	Digestive; burns toxins; spleen tonic; relieves muscle pain and congestion
Nutmeg *Myristica fragrans*	Pungent, astringent; hot; heavy; *tamasic* [pungent—reducing] -VK +P	Calms the nerves and gut; sedative; pain relieving; constipating
Parsley *Petroselinum crispum*	Pungent, bitter; heating; light; drying [pungent—reducing] -KV +P	Diuretic (without the loss of electrolytes); digestive; cleansing; tones the uterus and spleen; freshens the breath
Rosemary *Rosmarinus officinalis*	Pungent, bitter; hot; light; oily; sharp; *rajasic* [pungent—reducing] -KV +P	Digestive; antispasmodic; antimicrobial; antidepressant; expels mucus; supports nerves, circulation, mind, and memory
Saffron *Crocus sativus*	Pungent, bitter, sweet; hot; oily; light; sharp; *sattvic* [pungent—reducing] =VPK	Supports metabolism and nerves; blood purifier; rejuvenator; sedative; antispasmodic; antiseptic; aphrodisiac
Sage *Salvia officinalis*	Pungent, bitter, astringent; hot; light; dry; *rajasic* [pungent—reducing] -KV +P (in excess)	Digestive; removes mucus; diuretic; purifies blood; antibacterial; reduces hot flashes (drink cooled infusion)

8.   Fresh ginger is more soothing and building; dry ginger is more heating and penetrating.

Common Name *Botanical Name*	Qualities [vipāka] Effect on *Dosha* (V, P, K) "-" reduce/pacify; "+" increase/ aggravate; "=" neutral effect	Benefits
Thyme *Thymus vulgaris*	Pungent; hot; light; dry; sharp; *rajasic* [pungent—reducing] -VK +P	Digestive; antispasmodic; expels mucus; diuretic; promotes menstruation; antimicrobial
Turmeric *Curcuma longa*	Bitter, pungent; hot; dry; light; *sattvic* [pungent—reducing] -K +PV (in excess)	Reanimates and purifies digestion, blood, liver; anti-inflammatory; decongestive; anti-tumor; antibacterial; heals wounds

Water and Beverages

Āyurveda counsels that when thirsty, drink; and when hungry, eat. Drinking too much fluid when hungry, or before, during, or immediately after a meal, cools, dilutes, and dampens the digestive fires, weakens *vāta dosha*, increases phlegm and *kapha*, clogs the channels, and encourages weight gain. If the beverages are cold or iced, all effects are amplified. And carbonated soft drinks, concentrated in chemicals and sweeteners, further damage the pancreas, liver, and hormonal, immune, and skeletal systems, and feed inflammation and systemic degeneration.

Every day, fresh water is the best drink. Water fortifies the vital life-force *prāna*, supports tissue cleansing and lubrication, and lymphatic and immune functions, is largely considered *sattvic*, and, in the right amounts, helps to balance all *dosha*. In general, water is sweet to taste,

and cooling, plus, *Āyurveda* acknowledges the attributes of many different sources and types of water—rain water, well water, pond water, lake water, river water, spring water, tank water, dew water, snow water, seasonal water, distilled water, boiled water, warm water, and cooled water, plus tap water, bottled water, and filtered water. In general, chlorinated tap water is devitalized and likely to intensify *āma*, and fluoridated water may affect hormone and enzyme systems and hinder thyroid functions, making those exposed more vulnerable to illness and weight gain. Bottled water may have fewer chemicals than tap water, but lacks *prāna*, and can harbor plastic residues. Filtering water helps to remove toxic chemicals, but increases acidity; it is low in *prāna* but has more vitality than bottled water. Expose filtered water to the rays of the sun or moon to help cleanse and vitalize it for consumption. Today, fresh mineral water, in particular fresh spring and well waters, are considered highest in *prāna*. Mineral water is heavier, and spring water is lighter. Traditionally in India, water is stored in a copper vessel for between eight to twenty-four hours before drinking to kill present microorganisms, and assist the digestion and balance of all three *doshas*. Under the right circumstances, rain water is considered nectar, but perhaps these conditions have passed. In general, water that is boiled then cooled is considered light to digest, cooling, and does not increase mucus in the body.

Daily fluid requirements vary according to natal constitution, *dosha* imbalance, diet, physical activity, travel, work and living environment, and season. In general, those high in *pitta* need most water, and those with *kapha* dominance need least; diets high in dry, spicy, bitter, or astringent foods require more fluid supplementation; physical activity and travel needs liquid replenishment; artificially cooled and heated environments dehydrate the tissues and demand more fluids; as do hotter and drier seasons.

Ideally, daily beverages are enjoyed outside of meal times, an hour after eating, up until an hour before the next meal. Drinking water just before meals promotes weight loss (so may benefit heavy *kapha* types), and immediately after meals promotes weight gain (so may benefit thin *vāta*

types). During a meal, small sips of warm water are useful to liquefy solid foods, facilitate mixing with enzymes, and rinse the palate to enjoy full flavors. At other times, it can be best to drink larger amounts of water, dispersed by intervals, like our forefathers, rather than continuous sipping, which can confuse the body and encourage fluid retention. If dehydrated, however, continuous sipping promotes rehydration. At all times, drinking too much water leaches minerals and nutrients, dries out the kidneys and tissues, and reduces vital life-force.

Tea and Coffee

Prior to the seventeenth and eighteenth centuries, before tea and coffee became widely available, average beverage options for most Westerners ranged from dirty water, milk, beer, ale, cider, wine, and distilled liquor. (You can see where priorities have lain.) The introduction of tea and coffee provided a refreshing change that washes down a starchy meal, warms the body, and provides an energy boost in its wake. From an Ayurvedic perspective, both tea and coffee are generally bitter and astringent in taste. These flavors make tea and coffee immediately cooling, but heating and reducing in the long-term. Strongly fermented black teas can also be immediately heating.

Due to their bitter taste, astringent action, and presence of caffeine, both tea and coffee are drying, diuretic, and stimulating. These qualities dehydrate the tissues, create thirst, constipation, dry hair and skin, and *vāta* aggravation. In moderation they can benefit *kapha* types. Mild aromatic and green teas are sweeter, less fermented, and better for *pitta* types.

Bitter and astringent tastes assist digestion but are also last to be digested. Tea and coffee therefore are best avoided prior to and during eating. Their best application is as post-meal digestive. They may also help to reduce migraine headaches. Some Ayurvedic practitioners hold tea to be *sattvic*, although traditional specialists often forbade its use.

When tea, and especially coffee, are consumed daily, all *dosha* types are affected. The sharp, stimulating nature of caffeine encourages nervousness, anxiety, and insomnia. Caffeine disrupts the body's endocrine system, creating spikes and dips in blood sugar and energy levels, premenstrual mood swings, and an irregular menstrual cycle. In all *dosha* types, abstinence from caffeine can cure PMS and other hormonal and mood imbalances. *Vāta* types are most vulnerable. In pregnancy, caffeine enters the placenta but can't be processed by the developing fetus, and is best minimized, or avoided.

Compared to coffee, tea has about one third the caffeine and is better for daily use, especially for *vāta* and *pitta* types. Drinking tea with milk and warming spices such as ginger and cardamom helps to counteract caffeine's negative effects. After plucking, most tea leaves are not washed before drying, fermenting, and subsequent steeping, so choose organically grown tea and coffee varieties. And consider how the profits are distributed. If you drink coffee, choose freshly ground, or grind it yourself, as coffee readily oxidizes. Don't switch to decaf. Decaffeination requires strong chemicals.

Alcohol

The *Charaka Samhitā* describes eighty-four varieties of alcohol preparations made from various grains, fruits, roots, heartwoods, flowers, branches, and barks, plus sugar. Alcohol was adored by the gods, sustained Vedic rituals, and when taken appropriately, seen to support digestion, and produce energy, exhilaration, mental satisfaction, nourishment, virility, sleep, and rejuvenation. Fermented fruit wines were traditionally used as digestive stimulants, healing tonics, and as a vehicle for herbal therapies.

Alcohol is dominant in the fire element. Its qualities are sour, pungent, sweet, and bitter to taste, with a sour, heating *vipāka*. If not used judiciously, alcohol acts as poison. In excess it disturbs the liver, blood, pancreas, kidneys, and heart, destroys *ojas,* and aggravates all three *dosha.* In the mind, alcohol is initially *rajasic* and stimulating, then contributes the heaviness and delusion of *tamas.* If partaking of alcohol pay due regard to the type of drink; the foods eaten alongside; the season; the drinker's age, and state of *doshic* and mental balance.

Today's food choice decisions are no doubt more complicated than yesteryear. Food production is largely out of our hands, and the locus of growth, processing, and consumption are separated in space and time. Increasingly globalized food corporations suggest the marketplace is consumer led, while powerful conglomerates and multi-million-dollar advertising campaigns do much of the thinking for us. A confounding array of ready-to-eat products, clever marketing slogans, and cherry-picked research constantly redefine healthy food. All the while, large-scale monocrops and factory farming create artificial environments that are reliant on extensive inputs—many of them toxic chemicals that damage plants, animals, and ecosystems.

The foods we eat aren't created in isolation. Their production creates ripple effects across land, river, and marine environments. As well as *dosha* balance and digestibility, issues of ethics and quality suggest that biodynamic and organic farming methods that uphold or emulate natural habitats and practice regenerative farming methods are also better for plants and animals, better for Mother Earth, and better for us.

Regular Yet Flexible Eating

Eating to balance the *dosha* is a multifaceted affair that can be approached from numerous angles. We have considered many foods and food groups (and will provide further practical guidelines in Part II on page 129), but *Āyurveda* doesn't require that you rush to omit foods you've grown up with, are accustomed to, and feel somewhat attached to. When it comes to balancing *dosha,* *how* and *when* you eat can be just as important as *what* you eat.

When dietary habits are stable and advantageous, the digestion naturally prepares to receive food, and the metabolism is relaxed and efficient. Erratic eating, excessive eating, and late-night meals work against daily and digestive cycles. The body may manage irregular eating or overeating during early life, yet detrimental diets and hectic lifestyles, including too much travel and too many late nights, rob us of natural rhythms, weaken our adaptability, deflate the buoyancy of youth, confuse and tax digestion, accumulate *āma,* and imbalance the *doshas*. In contrast, appropriately structured meal patterns support all aspects of life, especially when maintained within a responsive approach that adapts to changing inner and outer circumstances. In *Āyurveda*, meal patterns occur within what is known as the daily routine or *dināchārya*. In order to help us be moderate in diet and recreation, methodical in the performance of actions, and regulated in sleep and wakefulness, establishing a daily routine is one of three primary *Ayurvedic* health and healing approaches. In creating a regular meal pattern within a daily routine, it's preferable to first work on structure and consistency, tailoring your approach according to *dosha*. Let's consider two central meal pattern features—meal frequency and size.

How Many Meals Is Ideal?

In hunter societies, as food became available it was eaten fresh, generally without reference to context or time. As environments changed, and food production and availability grew more regular, scheduled meal gatherings punctuated each day. Today our personal and social eating patterns have changed yet again. We are more mobile, work far from home, and live hectic lifestyles. Family mealtimes have eroded, and most individuals, including children, have continual access to widespread food choice.

When it comes to how many meals is ideal, Ayurvedic recommendations consider what's best for each constitution. The airy, variable nature of *vāta* constitution makes *vāta* types the most likely to eat erratically, avoid meal structure, and also the most likely to suffer. Managing *vāta dosha* is fundamentally about regularity, and reinstating natural cycles. Those with *vāta* constitution, and those managing *vāta* imbalance, generally benefit by eating three regular meals, that are small to moderate in size. *Vāta* types should take care not to overstretch the mid-meal interval. If lunch is on the light side, or dinner is late, an afternoon snack may be needed.

With their strong hunger and natural ability to digest, *pitta* types generally do well with three daily meals of moderate to large-size portions. Snacking is best avoided. And if digestion or metabolism feel heavy or sluggish, they benefit from light or skipped meals, and modified fasts.

For *kapha* types and those dominated by *kapha's* heavy, oily qualities, two daily meals suit best. If hunger is absent in the morning, listen to the natural appetite, and skip breakfast. Focus on a larger, nourishing brunch or lunch. Enjoy an early, lighter dinner. And avoid snacks. The heaviness of *kapha dosha* is readily pacified by eating smaller amounts, less frequently. Modified and liquid fasting can be beneficial. Part II provides more detailed dietary and fasting advice.

Mind Your Meal Size

In times past, the oral tradition of India advised that each meal should consist of thirty-two mouthfuls, and each mouthful should be chewed thirty-two times—one mouthful and chew for each tooth. Another way that Ayurvedic and Yogic practitioners consider meal size (that requires less counting), is to fill one part of the stomach with solid food; one part with moist foods or warm liquids; and leave the last part empty to provide space for the mixing of *doshas* and food. As a physical guide, the volume of the stomach can be likened to the size of both fists. Put together, one fist represents half of the stomach's capacity; make this the approximate size of a meal's solid food portion, with one quarter for soft/liquid foods, and one quarter free. This method allows for differences in body size. The right amount of food also depends on one's digestive capacity and *dosha* type.

Pitta types, with their hot digestive fire, often need to eat a little more, and are most likely to digest it well. *Kapha* types, with a lower, slower digestion do best with moderate amounts. *Vāta* constitution, with a lighter digestion, often experience an inconstant digestive capacity, and easily overeat or be satisfied with a small meal. Every meal, every day, if you care to listen, the body's subtle signals are real-time appetite guides to which you can attune. The right amount of food at each meal is ultimately that which you can readily digest.

According to *Āyurveda*, eating an appropriate *quantity* of food can be more important than the *qualities* of the foods consumed. Overeating taxes digestion and metabolism, and gives rise to heaviness and lethargy, hormonal imbalance, menstrual difficulties, weight gain, chronic disease, and premature aging. No species other than humans takes more than it needs, then still keeps on taking, even in surfeit. Yogic and Vedic texts describe overeating as a form of theft; stealing from other humans, animals, and Mother Nature.

Eating Patterns Must Also Be Flexible

History tells us there is no fixed way of eating. Humans have proven themselves capable of procuring, enjoying, and digesting a bountiful array of foods, in numerous contexts and settings. For nutritional health, the *right* food in the *right* amount is not a static one-size-fits-all approach.

Along with daily, monthly, and seasonal cycles, each body is different, and the body's requirements are constantly changing. We may want to be told "the way", but individual eating patterns must be flexible. Structure is necessary, but too much traps and inhibits.

The notion of *dietary responsiveness* involves observing ourselves (dominant elements, qualities, feelings, etc.), and our environment (dominant elements, qualities, cycles, etc.), and adapting food choice as different situations demand. A flexible eating pattern means that you do the following:

- Observe and question your existing eating habits, and avoid mindless repetition
- Use knowledge (theory) and personal experience (practice) to make informed choices
- Eat a variety of foods every day
- Be courageous enough to try new foods and, depending on the circumstances, say *yes* to some foods, and *no* to others
- Pay attention to the body for signs of hunger and satiation (fullness)
- Recognize that each day is different, and modify what you eat according to the external environment, and your current appetite and digestive capacity

- Don't rigidly deprive yourself of cultural or comfort foods that you truly enjoy. Eat consciously, and in moderation
- Do your best under ever-changing circumstances and feel content with, or at least accept and learn from your choices

Enjoying a structured yet responsive diet that supports your natal constitution will not happen overnight. Sustainable change occurs gradually, over weeks, months, and years, and is in fact, ongoing. While flexibility is always important, if your lifestyle is excessive or erratic it is best to focus first on establishing a regular meal pattern and becoming observant, before deviating from your plan.

When working in a holistic way, a positive change in one aspect of life is connected to and supports all others. Ultimately, there are many routes toward *dosha* balance, and each path can be unique. The more daily choices we orient in that direction, the greater the accumulated benefit. In Part II on page 129 we examine more practical aspects of choosing foods and eating patterns to balance every constitution.

CHAPTER 4

Stoke Your Agni (Digestive Fires)

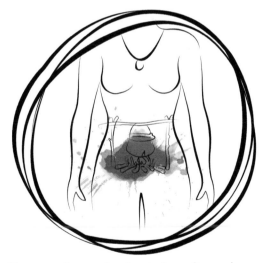

The agni, or digestive fires, burn in the gut, liver, and every cell in the body.

This chapter looks at the remarkable, essential process by which a little piece of Mother Earth becomes part of our bodily system. We explore the concept of *agni*—the digestive fires, and the extent to which each *dosha* type impacts the strength and characteristics of digestion. We look for signs of imbalanced digestion, and meet *āma*, or undigested toxins, that over months and years accumulate, and are seen by *Āyurveda* to underlie or contribute to almost all disease.

Today's nutritional science sees digestion as a mechanical, chemical, and microbial process. "Digestion" begins in the mouth, ends at the anus, and is basically confined to the gut. Chewing food and mixing in salivary enzymes begins the process, then the formed food-bolus travels to the stomach, then small intestine, where the bulk of digestion occurs. Here, strong enzymes and acids sever chemical bonds, reducing food to its basic constituents. From the middle to the end of the small intestine, nutrients are absorbed into the bloodstream and shunted to the liver for further processing. From the liver, nutrients enter general circulation. Everything that remains in the gut passes through to the colon, where it is worked on by bacteria. Water and some minerals are reabsorbed, and solid wastes form for evacuation which marks the end of the digestive process.

It is estimated that the physical body is made up of around ten trillion cells—and one hundred trillion single-celled microbes—the majority of which reside in the gut. Our physical being, it turns out, is not only wholly dependent on bacteria and fungi, we are largely bacteria and fungi ourselves. Known in the West collectively as the gut microbiome, this biomass helps to break down and digest food; manufacture nutrients; support brain and mitochondrial functions; assist immune functions, internal communication, and adaptation to external environments; detoxify and cleanse the body; and form a rich compost from digestive remains.[11] In the last decade, the discovery of the gut microbiome has shed new light on how digestion, mental health, and immunity are viewed.

Indeed, digestion is no simple task. From an Ayurvedic perspective, every meal involves complex interactions between the environment, foods, *dosha*, metabolism, mind, and behavior. And digestion is not confined to the mouth, stomach, and intestines. In the first digestive stage, food is split into digestible components and waste, before moving onto the second stage in the liver. Here, specific *agnis* work on each of the elements—earth, water, fire, air, and ether, releasing their respective qualities. A strong, functional liver is essential to perform this vital refinement to produce an excellent nutrient foundation for incorporation into all bodily tissues. If any aspect of digestion is inadequate or incomplete, the health of all tissues suffers.

Once processed, food's subtle constituents begin assimilation into each of the seven tissues in an inherently ordered manner—serum, blood, muscle, fat, bone, marrow, and reproductive cells. *Āyurveda* understands that the refined essence of food produced by the liver first becomes the nutritive fluid, serum. Serum in turn nourishes and produces blood; blood nourishes and produces muscle; muscle nourishes and produces fat, and so on; each level of digestion and metabolism becoming more subtle and refined. Each tissue is not just a substance; it is an essential support, a form of nourishment, and vital link in the chain.

The sequential process by which the tissues function and are nourished constitutes the third main digestive phase. Diffuse throughout the food body, fiery *agnis* reside in every living cell, continually cleaving, transforming, creating. As a group, these tissue fires form the largest digestive cooperative. The digestive process culminates with the expression of *ojas*, the most subtle and potentiated essence of food that powerfully vitalizes and nourishes the body and its immune and reproductive functions. A strong *agni* in the stomach and intestines is required for the two subsequent digestive stages to fulfill their role. In short, all three stages of digestion are required for the food body to be optimally nourished.

For *Āyurveda*, the digestive process extends beyond a transit through the gut. Digestion is seen as *the primary bodily process*, taking place in every living cell, a foundation that establishes the health of the entire organism. The digestive fires are life itself; one dies if the fires are extinguished. Through correct digestive functions, the *Charaka Samhitā* sees we are bestowed with energy, growth, strength, immunity, enthusiasm, perception, intelligence, heat, happiness, luster, and longevity. Balanced *agni* integrates all metabolic functions. Poor or incomplete digestion reduces the nourishment available to every bodily tissue, slumping the metabolism,

suppressing the immune system, and encouraging toxic buildup. Over time as tissues become burdened, they lose vitality and protection and become breeding grounds for disease.

In its treatment strategy, rather than target where the *doshas* end up (the location of the symptoms), *Āyurveda* targets the site where a *dosha* initially increases. As the home location of each *dosha* is in the digestive system (*vāta* dominates in the colon, *pitta* in the small intestine, and *kapha* in the stomach), these areas are often the starting point of *dosha* imbalance. This is an important reason why all *Ayurvedic* therapies consider the functions of the gut, and most treatments begin with the digestive system. To eat may feel imperative. But for the food body, the priority is that we digest.

Āyurveda sees that the digestive process proceeds based on three natural laws. *The law of selectivity* relates to the selection and rejection of foods. Just as a pigeon selects the most suited grains, humans should choose only suitable foods. Second, *the law of transformation* understands the digestive fires as a principle that processes and transforms foods into increasingly refined nutrition. The third natural law is *the law of irrigation* or *transmission*. As digestion proceeds, like irrigated water, food's essence is distributed throughout the body, drop-by-drop into increasingly subtle channels.

The Concept of *Agni*

In Sanskrit, the digestive fires are known as *agni*, the intelligent principle of fire. *Agni* is a heating, transformative energy that turns one thing into another without being altered itself. As fire transforms wood to ash, throughout the body the digestive fires convert food into new matter, without being changed themselves. From a biochemical perspective, *agni* relates closely to enzymes. Throughout our organism every metabolic function is facilitated by enzymes, the greatest concentration of which reside in the liver and gut.

Beyond a physical means, *agni* is a subtle concept. Along with the principles of *prāna* and *dosha*, *Āyurveda* views *agni* as a primary universal concept—the intelligent force that transforms one element into another, perpetuating the cyclic nature of life. The main qualities of the digestive fires are hot, sharp, and light. For conversion to be successful, *pitta's* heat, penetration, and light are required; plus, *vāta's prāna*, oxygen, and movement; *kapha's* lubrication and structure; and time. All factors must function well and in harmony. Too little fuel and the fires eventually go out. Too much fuel and the fires burn too hot, take on a life of their own, or are smothered.

In the body, the home of *agni* is the area around the belly and navel which includes the lower stomach, small intestine, liver, gallbladder, and pancreas. The fires of this region are the gateway between our external and internal world. Before digesting food, a balanced *agni* is a first-level defense against harmful foods, bacteria, viruses, and parasites by identifying which substances are nutritive and which are would-be intruders. A discerning *agni* chooses what to transform and accept into the cells, and where to apply protective processes such as vomiting, diarrhea, or burning up trespassers. That the intelligent *agni* recognizes and rejects intruders before they slip through a mucus membrane is a vital function of immunity and health.

For all pure and mixed *dosha* types, a balanced digestion looks different depending on the elements and qualities that dominate. But in general, expressions of balanced *agni* include a timely hunger and thirst, and absence of complaints such as reflux, bloating, heaviness, or constipation. Proper digestion is considered to have occurred when there is an absence of taste in the mouth; no bad taste or odor when belching; the eater feels light, enthusiastic, and vital; and well-formed stool, free from undigested particles, is eliminated between one to three times per day (depending on diet, constitution, and lifestyle).

In the food body the three *doshas* direct the functions of *agni*, and create our digestive nature. When the *doshas* are balanced, *agni* is balanced. Conversely, a fault in *agni* is also a fault in *dosha*. Along a spectrum, the belly's digestive fires tend toward four natural expressions: a penetrating digestion related to *pitta's* fire; a slow digestion related to cool, damp *kapha*; an irregular digestion related to the wind of *vāta*; and a *tridoshic* perfectly balanced digestion. Let's examine these now.

A Penetrating Digestion

A sharp, penetrating digestion supports a strong, fast digestive capacity that takes on most foods effectively. This expression of *agni* is most common in *pitta*-dominant types. A sharp digestion means that *pitta* people can be quick to feel hunger, and like to eat larger meals regularly. The elimination of wastes often occurs swiftly and copiously too. With an innately strong digestion, pure *pitta* and many dual *pitta* types can breeze through their twenties and thirties. However, in their late thirties and forties, poor habits tend to catch up.

If *pitta* becomes excessive, its hot, penetrating, spreading qualities transfer to the *agni*, bringing symptoms such as sour burping, acid reflux, abdominal tightness, nausea, and foul burning stools. Foods get "overcooked," and nutrition and tissues suffers. In the small intestine an overly sharp *agni* can kick-start inflammatory processes, including gastric ulcers, Crohn's disease, and ulcerative colitis.

A Slow, Low Digestion

A slow *agni* refers to an unhurried digestion that, when not overwhelmed, and given adequate time, eventually breaks down most foods. This type of digestion is mostly seen in those with *kapha* dominance and the heavy, stable attributes of earth and water. Pure *kapha* types seldom feel ravenously hungry. They may forget to eat, and can endure without food for the longest time. In a balanced self-regulating state, overeating at one meal creates a preference to skip the next meal, or eat simple and light.

In the kitchen, slow cooking is a superior culinary method that produces excellent results. When moderation is observed, those with a naturally slow digestion can enjoy robust health and life. Yet, when *kapha dosha* becomes excessive, cold, wet, heavy, dense qualities can dampen the digestive fires and mostly affect the stomach. In a depressed state, even frugal meals can cause fatigue, gastric heaviness, stuckness, and cravings for stimulants and sweets.

An Irregular Digestion

Irregularity in digestion reflects the mobile nature of wind. In a balanced state, *vāta's* movement is rhythmic, yet disturbed *vāta dosha* becomes variable. Natural appetites can vary from small frequent meals to one meal a day, yet the more variable digestion becomes, the more variable its expressions, from constant junk food cravings to absent appetite. As the digestive fires fluctuate, so does the ability to process each meal; a food digested one day brings cramps and bloating the next. *Vāta* aggravation can cause uncertainty whether to eat heavy food or light. Some meals are started, only to stop halfway.

From an Ayurvedic perspective, a variable digestion contributes to food intolerances and allergies, and irritable bowel syndrome (IBS)—common in *vāta* types disturbed by nervous tension. *Vāta's* changeable nature most affects the colon, producing gurgling, bloating, spasms, hard or painful or incomplete elimination, and fluctuations from constipation to diarrhea.

Perfectly Balanced Fires

Tridoshic types, born with an equal expression of all three *dosha*, are gifted with a perfectly balanced digestion, characterized by mild or subtle hunger, a silent digestion that effectively transforms food outside of conscious awareness, and the regular,

timely evacuation of waste. A balanced digestion also displays flexibility; according to what's available, the appetite adapts. Meals can be comfortably missed, and fasting is possible.

Imbalanced Digestive Fires

The digestive fires perform monumental functions but are ultimately subtle, sensitive, and vulnerable. For all *dosha* types, unbalancing forces include:

- *Prājñāparādha*, or mistake of the intellect, which leads to any of the following points
- Consuming foods with qualities that do not support the *doshas*
- Ignoring daily digestive cycles and seasonal cycles
- Overconsumption of any food
- Consuming too many cold foods and fluids, especially raw foods or iced drinks, especially at morning or night
- Consuming too many foods that are heavy or dry
- Consuming poorly cooked foods; polluted foods; incompatible foods
- Consuming new foods that the *agni* is not accustomed to
- Eating again before the previous meal is digested

- Drinking too much water or liquid just before, during, or after a meal
- Eating too little food
- Eating without attention, or during physical stress such as extreme fatigue, heat, cold, pain, or mental stress borne from worry, fear, anger, jealousy, hatred, greed, anguish, sorrow, and confusion
- Under- or over-activity
- Eating before exercising, swimming, or bathing
- Restraining natural urges
- Disturbed and irregular sleep
- Taking too many chemical medicines
- Excess alcohol, smoking, or recreational drugs

Āma: The Menace of Undigested Toxins

It has been said that *we are what we digest.* But actually, we are what we do, *and do not,* digest. In Sanskrit, the word *āma* means raw, uncooked, unripened; referring to substances that enter the body, yet don't undergo proper digestion. When the *agni* doesn't completely break down foods, the product is *āma.* Being improperly digested, *āma* is not readily assimilated into tissues. Nor can it always be evacuated from the body. Drop-by-drop, over weeks, months, and years, undigested *āma* accumulates. Rather than providing nourishment, undigested food becomes poison. Instead of feeding the body, *āma* inhibits normal functions and feeds pathogens and disease.

In the physical body, *āma* contains attributes similar to *kapha dosha*—heavy, dense, static, and oily, with a penchant to accumulate. As surely as a stagnant pond breeds mosquitos, stagnant pools of *āma* breed disease. Sluggish, fermenting *āma* nurtures bacteria, viruses, fungi, and parasites, which multiply beyond limits. As a force of decay devoid of intelligence, *āma* supports the organisms that eventually swamp the host.

In general, *āma* forms first in the gut as a result of low or irregular digestion. As *āma* builds, this tacky substance becomes glued to the intestinal wall occupying space devoted to nutrient absorption. The "villi," or finger-like projections lining the gut become clogged, impairing channels of nutrient absorption and systemic communication. As *āma* and pathogens assemble, they begin to eat into the gut wall. An Ayurvedic idiom states that "*āma* does not have legs." Unable to move around alone, to venture out of the intestines and journey into the blood and deeper tissues, it attaches to an aggravated *dosha.* Mixed with *dosha*, the cold, heavy, sticky qualities of *āma* mingle with the vehicle. *Āma* mixed with *vāta dosha* becomes colder, drier, crustier, and more adhesive. Mixed with *pitta dosha*, *āma* becomes an acidic, penetrating brew prone to drive inflammation. *Āma* and *kapha dosha* are even colder, heavier, and gooier, clogging the metabolism further.

In this piggyback arrangement, *āma* arrives in weakened tissues. Particularly vulnerable are systems, organs, and tissues that are already injured, overworked, inflamed, or somehow repressed or damaged. At susceptible sites, toxic residues slowly enter the channels and cells—obstructing, poisoning, settling in; moving the disease process deeper. By the time we feel symptoms, most diseases have been building for some time. If cleansing and rebalancing do not occur, conditions becomes chronic. In the process of disease, stemming from disrupted *dosha* and digestion, the buildup and infiltration of *āma* is seen as critical.

When the liver is exposed to contaminants daily it has less opportunity to remove waste, and eventually becomes exhausted. A compromised liver further enables toxins to accumulate. Plus, regardless of digestive capacity, some foods and activities are more likely to cause *āma*. In particular, old, refined, denatured foods; unseasonal foods; dining on foods that don't support our constitution; and eating more food than digestion can handle. For many, eating too much meat, too often, is problematic. Red meat can take up to three days to digest. That's seventy-two hours of semi-stagnation in warm, dark, wet environments—perfect conditions to breed putrid toxins. Plus, when solid wastes are not evacuated regularly, *āma* is quick to appear. Today the consumption of human-made pollutants including agrochemicals, toxic medications, heavy metals, and manufacturing residues can be added to the growing list of substances contributing to *āma*. If not regularly rested, cleansed, and rejuvenated, muck and inflammation build up, and the body malfunctions and prematurely ages.

Symptoms of *Āma*

As the gut loses function and digestion dwindles, the first indications of *āma* include feelings of fatigue, heaviness, weakness, and dullness. Having no zest for life. While not immediately life threatening, slow toxic buildup zaps physical energy and generates mental fog. Over time, joints become stiff, appetite wanes, constipation sets in, or headaches and migraines occur. While not outrightly unwell, a low-grade fever may linger, trying to burn up the toxic threat. Coughs and colds keep coming back.

Other signs of *āma* are loss of taste, and bad breath. If dental hygiene doesn't work, chances are you are harboring toxic waste. A thick, sticky tongue coating (especially first thing in the morning) is another strong clue. This coating reflects the qualities of the dominating *dosha*. *Āma* mixed with *vāta* presents a thin, dry coating that ranges from clear to cloudy, and sometimes dark or purplish in color. *Āma* mixed with *pitta* creates a moderately claggy yellowed coating. When mixed with *kapha*, *āma* on the tongue tends toward thick, white, and shiny. Another physical sign of waste buildup is lumpy cellulite on the hips and thighs.

In the gut, fermented toxins produce indigestion and painful bloating, cramping, and all kinds of noisy presentations. *Āma* in the colon makes feces feel sticky and stuck and produces heavy sinkers. Irritable bowel, diverticulitis, and colitis are other more overt presentations. As noxious wastes compromise the gut wall, toxins can migrate to the bladder, causing chronic urinary tract infections, and bacteria and proteins slip into the circulation unintended, known as leaky gut. Many allergic reactions and immune dysfunctions are also signs of *āma*. With its accrual, cellular communications fail, and the organism loses integration.

What Western medicine knows as atherosclerosis—sludgy fats and cells lining blood vessel walls—*Āyurveda* calls *āma*. Toxic buildup is seen as a primary cause of much heart disease. All chronic conditions, including arthritis and diabetes, are seen to be perpetuated and progressed by *āma*.

From an Ayurvedic perspective, health is sustained when the *doshas* are balanced, when the digestive fires are stable and strong, when all tissues function well, and wastes are regularly removed. In all of these areas, food is primary. If the diet is appropriate, and the digestive fires are strong, *āma* is not present. Even if *āma* is sometimes produced, a strong digestive fire ultimately burns up and removes unwanted toxins. *Agni* is opposed to *āma*. The presence of *āma* indicates that digestion is not balanced.

Today an increasing number of people suffer from poor digestive health. Day in, day out, foods and meals are too processed, too heavy, too much, too little, or otherwise too ill-suited. And we expect the body to cope. Within a seeming food abundance, mindless grazing of pickings on offer is a recipe for *āma* disaster. Unless born with an inherently robust constitution, or unless some effort is made, toxic, sludgy *āma* affects everyone.

Just as societies don't thrive in filthy, rotting environments, the body's tissues can't thrive in toxic grime. Only clean tissues can readily heal and support health. If the garbage is not removed, fumes and organisms take over, and decay sets in. To enjoy good health, the digestive fires must be stoked, and the rubbish must be removed. These principles, combined within an infinitely more local, modest food supply, remain relevant and universal.

Remove Toxic Buildup

Throughout the last century, thousands upon thousands of man-made chemicals and mountains of heavy metal residues have been released into the environment. We imbibe these never-before-seen substances in never-before-taken quantities, through the foods, beverages, and pharmaceuticals we consume; the air we breathe; the water we shower in; the clothes and personal products we wear; and other external sources. And whatever cannot be digested by the gut, detoxified by the liver, or safely eliminated accrues and weakens the entire system. If you experience one or more symptoms of *āma* accumulation, chances are tissue cleansing is required. Initiating health treatments without first eliminating underlying toxins can push poisons deeper, to eventually reemerge in a similar or different form. In a similar way, diseases suppressed by chemical medicines often reappear, while diseases eradicated by

detoxification treat the entire system and are cured at their source.

To expel built-up *āma* the food body needs support. First, we must reduce the toxins we take in. Prior to cleansing the system, it also pays to stoke the digestive fires. And after cleansing, the *dosha* must be balanced and digestive *agni* rekindled. Traditional Ayurvedic approaches to remove *āma* include active purification rituals involving massage techniques, herbal therapies, heat treatments, and *pañchakarma*— "five actions" that forcibly expel aggravated *dosha* and *āma* from the body. For thousands of years, *pañchakarma* treatments have been used to cleanse and purify the physical body of individuals with the time and wealth to take part. The five actions include cleansing the nasal passages and sinuses of excess *kapha* and *āma*; induced vomiting to cleanse the upper body of excess *kapha* and *āma*; purging the intestines and bowel of excess *pitta* and *āma*; enemas to cleanse the digestive tract and colon of excess *vāta* and *āma*; and other enema preparations to nourish and support *vāta*. Treatments are tailored to each individual's constitution and current state of health, and the season they are administered.

Before *pañchakarma* treatment, *Āyurveda* prescribes a light, simple diet, and the massage application of herb-infused oils plus heat to loosen and liquefy deeply embedded *dosha* and *āma*; internally, *ghee* may also be consumed. Ideally, one week of oiling precedes the cleansing of each of the seven bodily tissues. However, time can be scarce, and *pañchakarma* treatments are expensive. Yet, if too little time is spent preparing the body, receiving the cleansing treatments, resting, rejuvenating, rekindling *agni* and reintegrating back into daily life (including a *dosha*-balancing diet), the treatments can produce minimal results, fail, or promote adverse effects.

Pañchakarma therapies are strong in action, and best approached by robust individuals. This may sound counterintuitive, but in fact, *pañchakarma* is not a healing therapy. It is foremost for health maintenance and illness prevention, a seasonal or annual cleansing regime to prevent accumulated *doshas* and toxic buildup, thereby preventing disease. Since *kapha* qualities dominate in spring, a good time to cleanse *kapha* is just after winter, as the weather begins to thaw. To prevent diseases of *pitta* accumulation, the interim between spring and summer is a good time to cleanse. To manage *vāta dosha*, the interlude between summer and fall effectively reduces *vāta* buildup. In general, elimination therapy should not be undertaken in extremely cold, hot, or rainy seasons. A weak patient requiring treatment is first strengthened, and the illness appeased, before cleansing therapies are applied.

Systemic cleansing can (and often should) also be approached in more gentle, regular ways. We live in a polluted world; purification cannot be done once and then abandoned. Ongoing strategies include: minimizing your contact with toxins and hard-to-digest foods, balancing the *dosha*, strengthening the digestive fires, supporting the liver, keeping the bowels regular, consuming cleansing foods and fluids, appropriate fasting, moving the body, adequate sleep and rejuvenation, and intelligent use of the mind. In general, everyday cleansing is amplified when dietary and lifestyle choices occur alongside herbal treatments prescribed by a knowledgeable Ayurvedic practitioner or herbalist.

There have been cases where people suffering from illnesses including cancer, diabetes, heart disease, arthritic conditions, infertility, obesity, chronic fatigue, and a range of generalized, undefinable symptoms, unable to achieve health through a Western medical route, have found health through natural and adjunct cleansing therapies.[12] Among other benefits, detoxifying and fasting the body rests and revitalizes the metabolism and mind, improves sleep, resets and heightens the sense of taste, helps us break away from addictive behaviors, and increases our respect of food. After a period of cleansing, we have an opportunity to rebuild the food body as a more balanced, robust version. In the next chapter, this exploration begins with an overview of seven traditional methods to release excess *dosha* and lighten the body, plus Ayurvedic strategies to rejuvenate and rebuild the body with food.

CHAPTER 5

Langhana and Brimhana (Reducing and Building)

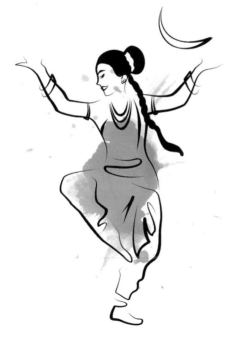

In *Āyurveda*, all therapeutic approaches and treatments belong to one of two broad classes: actions that reduce and lighten the *doshas* and tissues, known as *langhana* therapies; and actions that build and strengthen the tissues, known as *brimhana* therapies. The most intense form of lightening comes from the *pañchakarma* therapies, or the five actions used to forcibly flush excess *dosha* and *āma* from the body, discussed in Chapter 4 on page 90. Milder forms of lightening therapies alleviate and calm the *doshas* through fasting from food and kindling *agni*. In the realm of building treatments *Āyurveda* works in two main areas: rejuvenation and fertility. In this chapter, we consider how the five elements and foods can be used to lighten the tissues and alleviate the *doshas*, and how foods can be used to build and rejuvenate the body.

Lighten the Food Body

From an Ayurvedic perspective, the need to cleanse the tissues is common to all *dosha* types, while the need to lighten the tissues is more common in *kapha* types and those with *kapha* imbalance, and also sometimes in *pitta* aggravation. Today, increasing numbers of people are accumulating excess fatty tissue, known to *Āyurveda* as *kapha dosha* aggravation. *Kapha* is the *dosha* that manages the two heaviest, densest elements, earth and water, which together create adhesion and substance. Due to the natural dominance of these elements, those with *kapha* birth constitution tend to be of a bigger stature and gain weight easily. In other *dosha* types, too, once excess earth and water accumulate, their tendency is to adhere and attract more of their own. Plus, *kapha dosha* and *āma* share many qualities, and *like attracts like*. *Āma* conditions affect most people who need lightening therapies. Excess *pitta* can also drive tissue accumulation through an imbalanced *agni* and, when metabolic organs such as the liver and intestines become hot, fatty abdominal deposits are laid down to lubricate and protect the area against further heat.

Seven types of *langhana* or lightening treatments include:

1. Reducing water intake
2. Exposure to clean air and wind
3. Exposure to sunlight and heat
4. Kindling the *agni*
5. Digesting *āma* through maintaining the digestive fires
6. Fasting
7. Daily exercise

The first three approaches work directly with the elements. Reducing excess water intake (and other fluids) helps to dry and reduce excess tissue moisture. This is especially needed for *kapha* types and damp *pitta* types, and also involves avoiding foods that introduce water and oils such as sweet watery fruits and vegetables, tofu, nuts, seeds, and salts. The second and third approaches, exposure to wind and sunlight, introduce more air, ether, and fire elements into the body, helping to dry out and burn up excess tissues. Spending time in Mother Nature's drying winds helps to dry up excess *kapha* (but keep yourself warm) and cool and dry moist *pitta* types. Sunbathing introduces warm, light, sharp qualities that warm and dry *kapha* and gently approached can thaw cold *vāta*. We can also introduce more air into the body through pungent, bitter, and astringent foods, and also benefit from their long-term lightening effect. More fire can be introduced into the body through pungent and sour foods (salty foods should be used sparingly as they introduce water and their long-term effect is building; sour foods less so). Sweet foods should be avoided, but honey is an exception due to its special heating, lightening actions.

The fourth and fifth approaches which involve kindling *agni* and digesting *āma* are arguably the two most important daily therapies, and are discussed in detail in Chapter 8 (pages 115–127) along with the sixth approach—reducing food and fasting.

Most *kapha* earth and water elements enter the body through food. Lightening the physical body through reducing food is also a familiar Western approach. While most traditional cultures, including India, celebrate the plump, robust *kapha* form, Westerners admire the thin *vāta* form in women, and muscular *pitta* physique in men. Today—in a blink of time's eye—approximately one quarter of the world's population is considered overweight,[13] and a mind-boggling array of weight loss diets exist, most of which involve food restriction, calorie restriction, or a focus on specific macronutrients.

Take the Focus Off Calories and Weight

According to Western nutrition, to lose one pound per week, we must eat five hundred fewer calories per day, or burn off five hundred extra calories through physical activity. Yet, while the mind counts calories, the physical body doesn't relate to food in caloric terms, and this calculated notion rarely translates to the scale. Plus, thinking in calories reduces food to an abstract number— separate from whole foods, whole meals, and the wider environment. A focus on calories turns a slice of chocolate cake into a digit, while ignoring types and qualities of ingredients—natural eggs, whole sugar, real chocolate versus powdered egg substitute, artificial sweetener, and cocoa flavor. The latter contains fewer calories (and less taste), plus refined, artificial ingredients, foreign to our system. Concentrating on quantities of calories (and other nutrients), disregards the truth and complexity of the food body, ignores natural appetites, neglects the pleasures of eating, and obscures poor quality foods; a focus that suits the food industry. When the body is imbalanced, a focus on *weight* blames the problem on a singular symptom, and a focus on *weight loss* looks to arbitrary numbers—calories, pounds, BMI—when no problem, and no solution, exist in isolation. In contrast, *Āyurveda* thinks in terms of *dosha*, elements, and qualities, and focuses on rebalancing elements and qualities that are excessive through the strategy of *opposites reduce*, plus an emphasis on kindling the digestive fires, and cleansing the body of *āma*.

Be Active Daily

The seventh type of lightening therapy is activity. Today's technological developments in agriculture, transport, storage, and communications, plus the time-saving convenience of cars, supermarkets, and eateries allow us to move through each day and feed ourselves with little physical effort. At the same time, sedentary pastimes behind desks and computers, in cars and recliners, have amplified (and are often accompanied by snacks). But the body was built to move! We have a spine and hinged appendages. As a physical and energy system, everything must keep flowing: blood, lymph, cerebrospinal fluid, breath, *prāna*, and wastes. Appropriate physical activity kindles digestion and promotes strength, stamina, immune function, and resistance to discomfort and disease. It is well-established that regular exercise reduces the risk of high blood pressure, heart disease, diabetes, obesity, and countless common conditions. In the mind, regular activity promotes relaxation and lighter moods, reduces anxieties and neuroses, and encourages rejuvenating sleep.

To gain the most benefit from regular exercise, *Āyurveda* advises that we should start out slowly; exercise to the point where we feel warm, light, and energized—about fifty percent of total exertion. Choose activities suited to personal constitution, health, and age, and ensure deep, rhythmic breathing. In general, those with *vāta* constitution have a delicate skeleton and least physical endurance, followed by *pitta-vāta*. These constitutions benefit from regular, mild exercise that is gentle on bones and joints. Light, consistent training is preferable to sporadic exhaustion, and rhythmic exercise better than chaotic aerobics. Running and other heavy endurance activities stress and dehydrate light frames, and jarring activities lead to degenerating joints and arthritis later in life. Just after sunrise, *vāta dosha* enters a reducing stage of its cycle, so this is a good time to exercise.

Those with *pitta* predominance have a medium skeleton and physical endurance, and do best with exercise that is moderately effortful, yet not overly heating, exhausting, or competitive. At all times, and especially in summer, *pitta* and *pitta-vāta* types should guard against overheating and dehydration. Avoid the intensity of the sun, overly heated swimming pools, and bikram yoga. Take fluids before, during, and after physical activity.

Kapha types are generally blessed with strong bodies and stamina, and benefit greatly from daily exercise and intense aerobic and muscular movements that create heating, drying, stimulating, lightening effects to offset *kapha's* cold, moist, static, heavy nature. While many *kapha* types are drawn to comfortable lifestyles, lack of exercise is aggravating. Often encouragement is needed to get started, but once established, *kapha* types can increase effort and force, and stick with exercise routines and love it. Regular activity can be promoted by exercising with a friend, group, class, or team. *Kapha-pitta* types can also manage in strong physical pursuits, while those with *kapha-vāta* constitution have less strength and stamina.

Physical exercise should also take age into account. Prior to puberty, gentle, non-jarring exercise that helps to develop the senses and coordination is ideal. Set children free in yards, paddocks, parks, or down by the creek or pond. Create opportunities for them to develop physical reflexes, and hand-eye and motor coordination. Without these skills, physical movement can feel awkward and unnatural—in children, and as adults. Formerly inactive adults do well by making exercise a mindfulness practice. To build confidence naturally, begin with simple movements such as walking or basic yoga postures, and keep the mind on and in the body. When walking, bring the awareness just below the navel and consciously lead the activity from this center. Doing so disengages the mind and

introduces a grounding quality into movement. Observe new actions, skills, and experiences, and notice how they feel. Over sixty, the body naturally takes on more dry, light *vāta* attributes, and mild, non-jarring activities are best.

An active life should be a priority. All *dosha* types, of all ages, benefit by committing one hour per day to physical activity and awareness practices. Spring is a great season to get started. Find pursuits you enjoy and alternate your range of activities. Try new things and slowly progress as you go. As well as defined exercise, find ways throughout each day to move the body and generally be more active. In the realm of exercise and eating, *Āyurveda* advises no excessive exercise immediately after eating, but a short walk reduces heaviness, increases digestive ease, clears the mind and senses, and promotes longevity. All *dosha* types should avoid exercise when emaciated, or in the grip of intense hunger, thirst, anger, grief, fear, or exhaustion. Specific *dosha*-friendly activities are listed in Part II on page 143.

Lightening therapies are not prescribed to the extent that they go against physical strength and wellness. Indeed, mild lightening therapies are a lifelong mainstay. Applying the maxim *opposites reduce*, the lifetime diet for all *dosha* types is geared toward alleviating and balancing the *doshas*, regulating the digestive fires, minimizing *āma*, maintaining the tissues, upholding health and happiness, and preventing illness. When tissue and weight loss occur, this approach is no longer alleviating, but eliminating *kapha dosha* from the body, and potentially disturbing to *dosha* balance. Strong lightening and cleansing approaches, discussed further in Chapter 8 on page 115 are best used intermittently, according to individual constitution and need. Importantly, after intense or prolonged lightening treatments, before many therapies, and in youth and aging, *Āyurveda's* therapeutic approach also involves *brimhana* therapies to build and strengthen the tissues and constitution.

Build Up the Food Body

Over time, through continuous cycles of metabolism, the tissues wear and tear and functions become damaged and deficient. In *Āyurveda*, the goal of *brimhana* or building therapies is to uphold bodily intelligence, counteract natural deterioration, and support robust metabolism, mind and senses, virility, and longevity. Building therapies encompass rejuvenation therapies and virilization therapies. In particular, rejuvenation therapies aim to increase the amount and circulation of plasma in the body, the first of the seven tissues. Without abundant good quality plasma,

the healthy development of the six succeeding tissues is compromised, we lack contentment and vitality, and *ojas*—food's most subtle nutritive essence—is poorly formed and depleted.

For the food body, the principal nourishing, building therapy is food—primarily sweet, heavy, cooling, unctuous foods high in earth and water, such as wheat (barley if *kapha* is high), cow's milk, almonds and almond milk, other nuts, sesame, meat soups, grapes, unrefined sugars, and *ghee*. Toward their building goal, rejuvenating substances, including herbs, must be combined with digestive spices to boost their uptake and enhance circulation. Ensuring the digestibility of heavy revitalizing foods is a primary consideration, or *āma* is readily produced. Ideally, before undergoing rejuvenation, the digestive fires are stable and no *āma* is present, but this is often not the case. The best approach to rebuilding and rejuvenation is to take small amounts of heavy foods over longer periods (months), combined with digestives such as fresh ginger root (which promotes *agni*, is cleansing, and with a sweet *vipāka* is also building), and follow a *dosha* balancing diet and lifestyle, including appropriate exercise and adequate sleep. After the age of forty, *Āyurveda* recommends that everyone engage in some kind of rejuvenation therapy.

As well as the food body, *Āyurveda* understands that the mind needs rejuvenation, too. One key mental restorative is the quality of *sattva*, and reduction of *rajas* and *tamas*. To reinstate the mind's *sattvic* dominance, eating foods high in *sattva* and avoiding those that harbor *rajas* and *tamas* is an ideal start. Chapter 9 on page 153 explores the practice of *sattvic* eating and living. Other strategies to nurture and refresh the psychology include cultivating happy and peaceful emotions (while avoiding hot emotions such as anger, and withering emotions such as fear); herbal therapies; Yogic practices such as *prānāyāma* (breath expansion and control) and recital of *mantra* or healing sounds; and spending time in Mother Nature. In particular, frequenting natural forests and habitats is an excellent way to revitalize the life-force *prāna*, and balance and restore an ailing mental and physical constitution. We revisit these practices in Part II on page 154.

Another requisite to rejuvenate the mental and physical body is to follow a regular, supportive lifestyle and obtain adequate rest. The nature of activity is heating, stimulating, and reducing. To balance these actions we also need passivity, calm, and repose. During rest the physiological adaptations and benefits of activity occur, the mind and body cleanse and reset themselves, and rejuvenation and transformation happen. Allow the body and mind some rest!

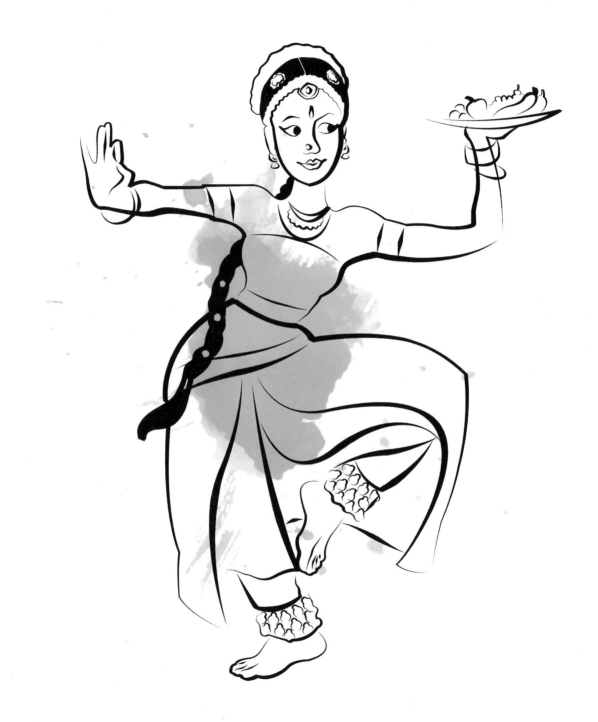

CHAPTER 6

Embodied Eating

Beneath star-filled skies, in mountains, forests, and plains, beside great fires and humble hearths, traditional cultures amassed vast compendiums of food knowledge and gave thanks for food's life-sustaining nourishment and pleasure. Fast forward to today, and most of the foods we eat are grown in faraway places, harvested, and transported through mechanized pathways across space and time. The food chain has become a series of convoluted linkages, mysterious processes, and implanted impressions. We are worlds apart from the animals that arrive on our plate as seafood and meat; with no concept of the beings involved in expediting our meals to the table—from other humans (farmers, transporters, traders, processors, technologists, manufacturers, sellers, cooks, and others), to the microscopic, and macrocosmic. We know little about the foods we eat, and seldom offer true observation or gratitude, let alone reverence or respect.

Eating to balance our constitution requires that we personally select more of some foods and less of others, depending on their elements, qualities, and tastes, and within nature's cycles. How we balance our unique *dosha* mix requires individual choices, but the concept and practice of embodied eating is relevant universally. Irrespective of *dosha*, we all experience hunger, are dependent on food, and (whether we are aware of it or not), accumulate its effects in the body. This chapter and its practical counterpart in Part II on page 159 counsel you to look, listen, and feel more deeply into your eating practices and experiences and the physical body itself. To use food as the vehicle to get to know the five universal elements, and work with their effects in the food body. To identify true hunger and interpret food cravings. To engage in conscious cookery. To elevate each eating experience and the foods we eat.

Eating is central to survival, and one of life's great delights, but for many, eating has become an automatic behavior—initiated without intention, occurring without awareness, continuing without control, operating efficiently, and with little personal effort. Instead of a dedicated pursuit, eating has become a conjoined activity—tacked on to driving, screen time, work, and mundane daily tasks. Food becomes secondary or tertiary. But automation is not how eating was intended. In the popular novel *Like Water for Chocolate*, Laura Esquivel quips, "Only fools and sick men don't give it [food] the attention it deserves."

Today, distractions hijack mealtimes. Through senses dulled by habit and familiarity, food plied with concentrated flavors that the taste buds effortlessly register are gobbled hurriedly in portion sizes we simply don't register. No conscious decisions or observant tasting enter into it. From an Ayurvedic perspective, mental and physical distractions while eating support *prā-jñāparādha*, or mistakes of the intellect, remove vital energy from the digestive fires, and disrupt

dosha balance, especially sensitive *vāta*. On the flipside, embodying the eating experience supports self-understanding, self-reliance, and intelligent choices; enhances digestion and assimilation; boosts physical, mental, and emotional satisfaction; reduces food dependencies; and helps balance the *doshas*.

Embodied eating relates to the Western concept of mindful eating that stems from the practice of mindfulness. In perhaps its deepest and original sense, the Buddhists call mindfulness a witnessing without judgement or preconception.[9] A mindful state involves keen observation, without expectation; an open attentiveness to the experience of life. A Zen proverb counsels: *When walking, walk. When eating, eat.* Don't *think* about being mindful or embodied, *be* embodied. Involve every sense in the total experience of food and eating, paying attention to appearance, textures, aromas, noises, flavors, qualities, how you eat, and how the experience merges with your food body.

Eating is fleeting. For the time you eat, stop reliving the past, don't worry about the future; entirely surrender to the eating experience. The Indian mystic known as Osho or the Bhagwan Sri Rajneesh, said:

While you are eating, then let there be only eating and nothing else, then let the past disappear and the future too; then let your whole energy be poured into your food. Let there be love and affection and gratitude toward food. Chew each bite with tremendous energy and you will have not only the taste of the food but the taste of existence, because the food is part of existence. It brings life; it brings vitality, it brings prāna. It makes you tick on; it helps you remain alive. It is not just food. Food may be the container: life is contained in it. If you taste only food and don't taste experience in it, you are living a lukewarm life . . . [9]

Āyurveda sees food as a sacrifice from the universe, an offering to our digestive fires; an act that should involve attention, gratitude, and reverence.

Like the need to breathe and reproduce, the need to eat and drink is too important to be left to chance. As well as observing the act of eating and reverence for food, embodied eaters also notice digestion; listen to the body's wisdom of physical hunger and satiety; and witness how they feel before, during, and after a meal. After the unconscious urge to breathe, hunger is a primary driving force. Both Ayurvedic and Western sciences understand that hunger is driven by internal and external factors. From a Western perspective, two pleasure systems are involved in feeding. A premeal system drives a sense of expectancy and reward, stimulating appetite and eating. During and after food, a second pleasure system releases happy hormones, known as endorphins, that relax the body, lighten the mind, and generate short-term feelings of reward and contentment. Now, with such ready access to food, through little or no effort, we can be "rewarded" time and again.

Western science also holds a range of hormones and chemical transmitters internally regulate short—and long-term hunger, operating between the gut and brain. Hormones by the name of insulin, ghrelin, neuropeptide Y, agouti-related protein, and orexins A and B promote hunger and eating. While substances known as cholecystokinin, glucagon-like peptide-1, leptin, peptide YY, pro-opiomelanocortin, and alpha-melanocyte-stimulating hormone carry messages that reduce hunger and oppose food consumption.[15]

---

9   From a spiritual perspective, mindfulness is a stepping-stone to the Divine. Before responding to anything, Gautama Buddha taught his followers to be mindful; to be aware, and witness clearly, without bias.

But our appetite control is biased, geared to stimulate hunger more readily than suppress it. Hunger is a powerful survival tool, an insurance policy against starvation.

Rather than begin in the mind, true hunger is a bodily sensation that turns into the thought, *I'm hungry*. From an Ayurvedic perspective, hunger is driven by the *agni*, or digestive fires. When the preceding meal has been fully "cooked," and the controlling *doshas* are balanced, hunger lets us know that the digestive fires are ready to receive more food. But hunger is also misunderstood, misinterpreted, and mis-imagined. Today, natural hunger and appetite rhythms are disrupted by:

- Emulating peers or significant others
- Allowing commercial interests to sell us food
- Eating junk food
- Assigning emotional roles to food
- Being on a fixed diet, or "see-food" diet
- Stress
- Erratic lifestyles
- Inadequate sleep
- Constantly catering to the likes and needs of others, without acknowledging our own preferences and needs
- Children given too little autonomy in hunger and fullness decisions

In Part II on page 159, we explore how to embody eating within the context of regular, supportive practices to bring us back in touch with the body's wisdom, and reacquaint ourselves with true hunger and satiation.

In traditional cultures, all adults were involved in some aspect of food procuring, growing, preparing, and cooking, and the children observed and pitched in. Today, food growing, gathering, processing, and preparing are largely outsourced to others. Our most direct involvement is eating. Nowadays, hunting and gathering are rare and problematic activities, and if we don't have the time or resources to grow our own food, the best (and perhaps only) place to start relationship-building with food is in the kitchen, or when presented with a plate.

Ingredients prepared with knowhow, care, and gratitude introduce new energies to foods. In the alchemy of cookery, many cultures have considered the physical and moral qualities of the people preparing foods, understanding the cook contributes to the food, and these energies become embodied in the consumer. Hopefully we have all experienced the upliftment of a meal prepared with joy, generosity, and nurturing intentions. While the work of an angry, frustrated cook delivers a dispiriting blow. Food can carry love or loathing into the system. For this reason, the *sadhus* or wandering holy men of India traditionally only ate meals they prepared themselves. Ideally, food is handled with gratitude, respect, and intentions to nurture the needs of the eater. In cooking, as in life, we can be a conscious contributor.

Āyurveda understands that natural foods are a gift from Mother Nature, a piece of the universe created to sustain earthly life. There is also a certain violence in raising, killing, and processing the plants and animals we eat. Consciously appreciating and acknowledging the nature of eating increases its benefits, and reduces its negative effects on us as individuals and on the wider cosmos. Creating a relationship with each meal and offering heartfelt thanks raises food's energies, enhances our personal and collective vibration, and elevates our eating experience and encounter with life.

The more we embody the eating experience, the better equipped we are to also realize when something's *not* right—when feelings rise in the gut, chest, mouth, or throat; when a food or act does not suit us. Many decisions to eat or drink only last a moment. Being present to a feeling or urge—even if it doesn't change our behavior—opens a doorway of choice. Rather than react and eat out of habit, conscious, embodied eating develops flexibility of choice.

No doubt, the current food environment does not support embodied eating, especially when we eat food in public. All inner events exist in deep interdependence with our social surroundings, and the ecosystem, including soils, water, air, animals, and plants, as well as daily and cosmic cycles. To genuinely embody eating, we must look deeply into our food-related practices and experiences and identify the truth of our personal and worldly circumstances. In doing so, we advance our relationship with our self, the foods we eat, and the world we inhabit, and know our unique place within it. In Chapter 10 on page 159 we explore many components of, and ways to approach, embodied eating.

In summary, a balanced diet and lifestyle are organized and regular, yet flexible and responsive to inner and outer change. Key principles of Ayurvedic nutrition understand that:

1. We are an elemental part of Mother Nature
2. Food builds the food body, and the foods we eat and the ways we eat them contribute to either health or disease

3. The key to balanced health is eating to balance one's unique *dosha* or constitution
4. The *agni* or digestive fires play a fundamental role in health, and must be kept alight
5. *Āma* or undigested toxins are a primary force underlying disease and must be minimized
6. To balance our unique constitution within daily life:
   - Pay attention to the wisdom of the food body
   - Pay attention to the environment, and live in accordance with natural cycles
   - Minimize foods high in the qualities you already have (*like attracts like*)

- Choose foods with complementary qualities (*opposites reduce*)
- Eat natural, fresh, seasonal foods that include all six tastes in harmonizing proportions
- Create regular eating patterns that are responsive and adaptable
- Consider how you treat, eat, and relate to food
- Cultivate complementary lifestyle activities

With this foundation, let's now begin *Living Āyurveda*. Part II focuses on putting these key principles into action.

PART II

Living Āyurveda

Over the ages, and today, people have offered many different principles and beliefs to help us fathom personal and worldly meaning, and improve our health and well-being. But ideas and information remain concepts only and are of no practical value unless they are practiced and lived. True understanding and benefit come when applicable knowledge is consolidated through personal first-hand experience.

Āyurveda is not a set of rigid rules. It is a living science and wisdom; a path where each individual can fully involve themselves in healing imbalance that afflicts them, and maintaining robust health. Along the path of self-healing, *Āyurveda* encourages people to seek expert advice, then consolidate understanding through personal observation, awareness, and experience. In this way, theory informs and regulates practice, and practice informs and expands how we relate to theory. Personal application brings information and discourse to life. The Indian traditions of *Āyurveda*, yoga, and *Tantra* have always flowed between the twin shores of theory and practice.

Today it's possible to take little personal responsibility for the foods we eat. But from an Ayurvedic perspective, eating and food choice shouldn't be influenced by cherry-picked scientific studies, big corporations, or what's at arm's length in the store. Eating is ultimately a *personal* affair that takes a little time and commitment. By paying attention to foods, to the eating experience, and to food's effects, we can better understand their qualities and whether they suit us or not. We may hear about mangoes all our life, but until we smell its fragrant aroma and experience its complex sweet-sour taste and dense, juicy flesh in the body, and its heating effects if we eat too many, we never really *know* mango. Taking responsibility for our choices means we may sometimes not get it right. Yet through experience, doubt is removed, and faith in our capability grows.

Part II: Living *Āyurveda* is about putting the principles of Ayurvedic nutrition discussed in Part I into practice. Only then can we consolidate helpful knowledge, and truly reap the rewards. Holistic approaches understand that change in one area is connected to, and affects everything else. With this in mind, undertaking change in any area can help to balance the whole. But perhaps the best place to start, the most fundamental, is to reconnect with Mother Nature, the divine principle of material creation, of which we are part.

CHAPTER 7

Embracing Mother Nature's Cycles

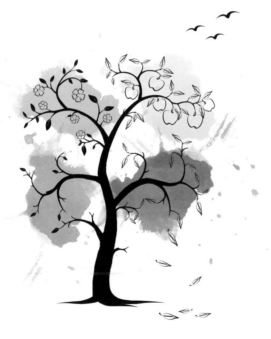

Āyurveda sees that material life arises from the force of Mother Nature through the potencies of *sattva*, *rajas*, and *tamas*, and the mix of the five great elements that generate the daily and seasonal cycles, and the larger cycle of life. Today, led by historically male-dominated cultures, expanding urban environments, and decreasing natural habitats, many of us are nature deprived and out of touch with the reality and subtlety of Mother Nature's cycles. Yet, by paying attention to, and aligning ourselves with natural laws, forces, and elements we better understand ourselves and can work in harmony with Nature, rather than against the cosmic flow.

Harmonizing with Seasonal and Daily Cycles

Ayurvedic nutrition understands that we exist in deep interdependence with our surroundings.

We are connected to the plants and animals with whom we interact, and the local and cosmic spaces we occupy. Eating to balance the *dosha* requires we take this interdependence into account, inclusive of the continual influence of daily and seasonal cycles.

As the dominance of atmospheric elements change, so change the seasons, our physical body, our ease of staying in balance, and our ability to tolerate certain foods. To what extent each season affects us depends on our personal elemental mix. If the season brings qualities opposite to our constitution, the *dosha* are naturally pacified and less prone to aggravation because *opposites reduce*. Spring's warming, moist qualities counter the cold, dry attributes of *vāta dosha*; the chill of winter cools hot *pitta* fires; and dry, windy fall helps to lighten oily, stable *kapha*. When supported by opposite ecological qualities we may tolerate foods and activities that at other times provoke imbalance.

Correspondingly, when the qualities of the season are similar to our own, *like attracts like*, and we take on more already dominant elements. At these times, eating for *dosha* balance by applying the principle *opposites reduce* becomes especially important. Throughout fall and early winter, the climate can be cold, dry, and

changeable. Pure *vāta* types, mixed *vāta* types, and those with *vāta* aggravation need to take extra care to choose warm, moist, nourishing meals at reliable intervals. In the annual heat of late spring and summer, pure *pitta* types, warm dual types, and those with *pitta* excess can more readily overheat, and should consciously choose cooling foods to restore and maintain balance. In the cold, wet months of late winter and early spring, *kapha* types, *kapha* dual types, and those with *kapha* imbalance should choose warm, dry, light, stimulating foods to protect against excess mucus buildup. Eating in accordance with *opposites reduce* represents the advice for all *dosha* types, but is most important in *like* seasons.

For dual *dosha* types, eating with the seasons makes particular sense. When the climate is aggravating for one *dosha*, choose pacifying foods. When the seasons change, and the other aspect of the constitution is challenged, focus on choosing foods with qualities *opposite* to the vulnerable *dosha*. *Pitta-vāta* constitution can eat to pacify *pitta* in spring and summer, and *vāta* in fall and winter. *Pitta-kapha* types can eat to cool *pitta* from late spring, through summer to early fall, and support *kapha* through winter to early spring. *Kapha-vāta* constitution can eat to pacify *kapha* in late winter and early spring, pay more attention to *vāta* in fall and early winter, and in summer choose according to whether the elements of water or air dominate alongside heat. All *dosha* types, but especially *vāta*, must be alert to prevent imbalance during the changeable weather between seasons.

Within each day, there's also a cycling of elements and qualities. Mornings are cooler and damper; middays hot; afternoons drier and airy; and evenings becoming cool and moist again. Over every day-night cycle, each *dosha* moves through stages of peak and decline. While one *dosha* is peaking, another is declining, and the third is on the rise. Every twenty-four hours each *dosha* has two peak phases, followed by stages of relaxation and regain.

In the cool, damp of early morning, *kapha dosha* dominates. From midmorning, the sun warms and *pitta* reigns. The drier, cooler afternoon cycles to *vāta*. With dusk, *kapha* returns. Over the midnight hours, *pitta* works to complete digestion. And in the predawn hours, *vāta dosha* busily transports wastes.

It is during each *dosha's* peak phase that *dosha* aggravation most readily occurs. *Kapha dosha* is most readily aggravated in the cool damp of morning and night. This is the most important time to minimize sweet, salty, oily, cold, heavy *kapha*-aggravating foods, and why *kapha* types (and ideally all constitutions) should avoid eating late at night, especially cold, heavy foods such as dairy. In the heat of the day, *pitta* types should minimize heating tastes and foods. A salty, spicy meat dish for lunch is inviting *pitta* aggravation, as is strenuous physical activity. In dry windy afternoons and cool early evenings, *vāta* types are particularly vulnerable. At this time, they should take extra care to avoid dry, light, cold foods and elements; instead focusing on warm, moist, dense options. The time of day that disease symptoms tend to get aggravated provides a clue which *dosha* is responsible. When a *dosha's* dominance continues outside the natural *dosha* cycle, if not corrected, seeds of disease are sewn.

The daily *dosha* cycle is associated with a daily digestive cycle. While *kapha dosha* dominates from dawn (6:00 a.m.) until midmorning (10:00 a.m.), it's every body's time to cleanse. To support the liquidation and removal of wastes and excess *dosha*, breakfast can include foods that assist elimination such as fruit, warm whole grain cereals, and herbal teas. From 10:00 a.m. to 2:00 p.m. when the sun is at its peak, *pitta's* digestive fires are strongest and the main meal can be eaten. As the day and body cools, the digestive fires weaken and by dusk have lost their bite. Evening meals should ideally be eaten early and kept light.

Understanding the daily *dosha* cycle helps to better plan each day, to tailor what to eat—or not—and when to act—or not—as each case may be. Ayurvedic nutrition involves paying attention and responding to the elements and qualities that dominate in the physical body and outside over each day and season, and as these factors change over time. As the seasons change, so do the natural ripening of fruits and vegetables—another important aspect of seasonal eating.

Eating Seasonal, Local, and Fresh

The commercial production and transport of food has increased many people's access to an extraordinary range of fruits and vegetables. Today we can make food choices independent of locality, geography, and season. We can pick up asparagus grown in Argentina, mangoes from the tropics, or crunch on an apple regardless of season. Seemingly abundant petroleum resources, transport efficiencies, and modern technologies render many foods readily mobile commodities. This global food market seems expedient, and seems to give us what we want, but a globalized food system mostly suits business and politics. In reality, human beings and their communities can only thrive when most

food needs are met locally. The most long-lived humans, in the earth's "blue zones," subsist on local, seasonal produce, within purposeful family and community-oriented surroundings. *Āyurveda* emphasizes food choices that are local and seasonal, with an emphasis on cultural and ancestral influences. Your food body is attuned to these foods.

Only locally grown fruits and vegetables have the chance to ripen naturally. Foods grown and ripened in their natural habitat and season have the opportunity to develop their full taste potential, be readily digestible, and most deeply nourish the body. When seasonal fruits and vegetables are eaten within annual cycles, the *agni* recognizes these phases, and tends its fires accordingly. Plus, eating seasonally and locally greatly simplifies the food chain. Foods endure less time in the travel, refrigeration, gassing, and storage processes. Choosing locally grown produce conserves natural resources and is a vote for the local biodiversity and economy. Plus, eating with the seasons represents the first and truest meaning of variety.

Local, seasonal foods are also the freshest option. Fruits and vegetables grown and allowed to ripen in natural ways are minimally processed (skinned and cooked, if necessary), and can be consumed in close time-space proximity. *Āyurveda* understands fresh foods are naturally sweeter, cooling, moistening, and *sattvic*, and counter inflammation and acidity. They are also high in the life-force *prāna*, and inherently vitalizing. As foods age they become more sour and bitter, heating, drying, *tamasic*, inflammatory, acidifying, and lifeless.

Today, *fresh* is a relative concept. The distinction fresh is applied to produce that has been plucked unripe, imported, gassed, and cold-stored. Enthusiastically adopted by marketing campaigns, we are conditioned to the idea that fresh foods are available year-round, and can sit on supermarket shelves, and in pantries, fridges, and freezers. To support eating seasonal, local, and fresh, you can do the following:

- Get educated about the different fruits and vegetables that grow locally and seasonally in your area. Explore farmer's markets. Ask food sellers for locally produced foods.
- Plant indigenous fruit trees, and grow your own seasonal produce.
- Check "country of origin labeling" (COOL). While not mandatory globally, some countries place a requirement on food manufacturers to indicate where a food is grown. Unfortunately, the COOL label is considered too complex for processed, multi-ingredient products.
- If you don't have access to foods grown locally, still choose foods grown within the current season. An exception to this is grains and pulses, which become drier and lighter to digest one year after harvest.
- Hand-select your fruits, vegetables, seeds, and nuts. Allow fruits to ripen at room temperature in natural light. Store fresh produce in a cool, dark, airtight place. Shop little and often.
- Wherever possible choose organically produced foods. Particularly organic foods grown using regenerative techniques that focus on soil health. This buoys food's nutrient density, microbial diversity, and digestibility, and supports the health of ourselves and Mother Earth.
- Plan ahead. If you can't always access fresh food, carry it with you.

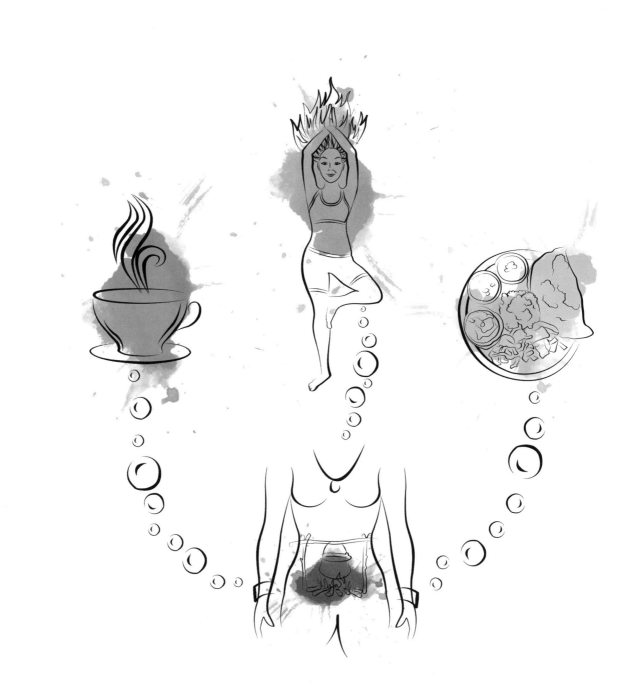

CHAPTER 8

Stoking Your Digestive Fires

The digestive fires govern the process by which a little piece of Mother Earth becomes part of us, a principle of transformation that takes place in every living cell. The digestive fires transform life, and are intelligent life itself; the foundation of energy, growth, strength, metabolism, immunity, happiness, and longevity of our entire organism. The primary qualities of *agni* are warm, sharp, and light. The quality of *light* is associated with the luster and brightness of fire, and also its lightening, reducing, purifying nature.

In contrast, poor or incomplete digestion causes heaviness and fatigue, flags the metabolism, suppresses the immune system, imbalances the mind, and creates *āma* or undigested toxins that underlie or contribute to almost every ailment.

Imbalanced digestion also reduces the nutrients we can extract from food and the nourishment available to every bodily tissue. Two people may eat the same meal, but their bodies do not receive the same nutrition. It all depends on the food body's ability to digest and assimilate.

To enjoy balanced *dosha* and balanced health, for the food body the priority is that we digest. This chapter presents strategies to kindle the *agni* and support digestion, followed by an exploration of ways to eliminate *āma*, or toxic buildup.

The Medicine of Negation

The medicine of negation is a powerful dietary tool. To strengthen digestion the best place to start is to stop doing things that bring imbalance. Rather than thinking in terms of what to eat, think first in terms of what is best minimized or avoided. The knowhow of the *no* is self-empowering. By saying no to foods, we are saying no to the momentum that supports the habit or calls it into being. Saying no also subdues the mind and helps to reestablish the voice of the body. Rather than take foods, herbs, or medicines that we think or hope are good, it's often better to take and do nothing, and not overburden the body. If in doubt of what to do, move toward the positive by working from the negative; remove what is problematic first. All *dosha* types can apply the medicine of negation to support the digestive fires by not consuming the following:

- Too many foods and tastes with dominant qualities similar to your own (*like attracts like*)
- Too much food or too little food at mealtimes, according to body size and constitution
- Cold foods and fluids, especially iced drinks that put out the digestive fires. And too much water or liquids just before, during, or after a meal
- Dry foods that take moisture from the digestion and body (especially *vāta* types)
- Heavy foods, for example anything deep-fried, that the body has little chance of fully digesting

- Unseasonal foods, poorly cooked foods, too many food combinations, and incompatible foods in one sitting
- Foods that the *agni* is not accustomed to, such as imported foods and chemically grown and processed foods
- Sterilized and long shelf life food that is inert and anti-life

We can also apply the medicine of negation to our actions by consciously not consuming meals during the following times:

- Counter to the daily digestive cycles
- Before the previous meal is digested
- When we are distracted from our food and ourselves
- While very hot or cold or in pain
- While experiencing extreme fatigue, stress, worry, nervousness, fear, anger, jealousy, hatred, anguish, or sorrow
- Immediately before exercising, swimming, or bathing
- In the hour before undertaking mentally challenging endeavors
- During a partial or full lunar or solar eclipse

We can also say no to meals for a day or two, and rest and rejuvenate the digestive fires through fasting (discussed shortly). Other things we can say no to include:

- Allopathic medications that silence the messenger, allowing disease to continue and spread. Such as antacid compounds and protein pump inhibitors for heartburn and reflux that, ironically and disastrously, further derange digestion by suppressing digestive acids and enzymes, driving toxins deeper, supporting constipation and weight gain, and reducing immunity—while the foods and behaviors underpinning the issue remain.
- Agricultural pesticides such as glyphosate that kill natural soil and plant microbes; the use of broad-spectrum antibiotics; routine pasteurization and sterilization of food; too many germ-killing fluids for personal sanitization and home-based disinfection. All first-rate ways to ruin the gut ecology.
- Lifestyle choices, including alcohol, smoking, and irregular sleeping patterns
- Under-activity
- Over-activity (including sexual)
- Restraining any of the thirteen natural urges
- Harmful activities and relationships

In their treatment of *dosha* imbalance, Ayurvedic practitioners generally proceed in a certain order: First, the cause of *dosha* imbalance must be removed. In accordance with the law of cause and effect, if you do not want an effect, remove the cause, where possible applying the medicine of negation. Second, excess *dosha* and *āma* must be eliminated through cleansing and purification. Third, the *dosha* must be balanced, and the digestive fires rekindled. Fourth, rejuvenate the tissues and system. Regaining a healthy digestion often takes three to twelve months, depending on the extent of the imbalance, the body's and mind's adaptability, and whether or not the environment is supportive.

As a starting point of treatment, the medicine of negation may sound straightforward—and can be—but physical and mental habits are often barriers to be crossed. With attention, the mind can adapt and redirect behaviors—weaning off former favorites and acclimatizing to new culinary experiences. But even with attention, biological adaptation occurs at the pace of Mother Nature—weeks, months, years, or generations. (We explore the art of habit change in Chapter 11 on page 185.) While applying the medicine of negation, steps to directly support the digestive fires include:

- Eat foods with tastes and qualities that balance your constitution (*opposites reduce*)
- Prioritize fresh, seasonal, well-prepared food
- Include foods that stimulate the gut and liver *agnis*, such as pungent mustard greens, horseradish, kohlrabi, watercress; bitter cabbage, broccoli, and Brussels sprouts. Before eating, chew on a thin slice of fresh ginger marinated in a few drops of lemon juice or pinch of rock salt.
- Include fermented foods such as yogurt, pickles, kefir, sauerkraut, kimchi, tempeh, apple cider vinegar, soy sauce and tamari, and other foods that feed the gut flora such as dandelion root, burdock root, yakon root (a sweet potato), Jerusalem artichoke, onion, leeks, garlic, ginger root, and chicory root teas.
- Cook and make teas with digestive spices such as fresh ginger, turmeric, cumin, fennel, cardamom, black pepper, basil, rosemary, bay leaf, mint, and lemon balm. For guidelines for each *dosha,* see Chapter 9 on page 143.
- Participate in regular physical activity, relaxation, and meditation and nurture a breathing pattern that is rhythmic and deep.

- Perform yoga practices that unblock physical and subtle channels, and awaken and balance the breath and digestive *prāna,* including physical postures, breathing exercises, *mudras* (hand gestures), and concentration, visualization, and meditation. We return to these ideas as we go.

Another important way to support digestion is to ensure the bowels are regular. When the bowel is sluggish, more toxins are created and absorbed. We visit the bowels in some detail in Chapter 10 on page 170. Kindling the digestive fires supports the second step of treatment, to cleanse and purify the system. As digestion improves, the *dosha* become more balanced, and less *āma* is produced. A strong *agni* can also identify and burn up stored toxins, but help is often required. Let's embark on the *how to* of burning up and removing toxic waste.

Eating to Remove *Āma* (Toxic Buildup)

Over time, toxic *āma* accrues in the gut, infiltrates vulnerable tissues, and weakens the entire system. The main indications of *āma* are persistent fatigue; smelly sinking stools; a furry tongue coating; being sick all the time, among others, discussed in Chapter 4 on page 88. Experiencing one or a collection of *āma*-related symptoms indicates the digestive fires need boosting, and tissue cleansing and detoxification is required. From an Ayurvedic perspective, regular cleansing is the best way to prevent disease and to help many diseases heal.

In *Āyurveda*, the best-known cleansing therapies are the collection of five strongly reducing actions, known collectively as *pañchakarma*, discussed in Chapter 4 on page 90. So too, *āma*-reducing strategies can be approached in more gentle ways, and followed for one or two meals; an entire day; two or more consecutive days; a week; a few weeks; or a month or more at a time. In general, *vāta* types should choose gentle options, and think in terms of a few meals or days, or follow a cleansing diet for one day per week or fortnight. Robust *pitta* types might follow a mild cleansing diet for a few days, a week, or several. Those with *kapha* dominance can tolerate and benefit from stronger *āma*-reducing strategies, up to three or four months at a time. For many, after a lifetime of unhelpful habits, it can take months of daily or weekly detoxification to rid the deeper tissues of accumulated deposits.

In general, the best time to undertake an extended period of cleansing is the junction of seasons, especially the end of summer and beginning of spring. In hot climates, cleansing can be initiated year-round. In winter and cold climates, cleansing diets are best avoided. At all times, if the body is detoxified too fast or too long, symptoms can occur such as persistent headaches, fainting, complete lack of energy or motivation, loss of appetite, nausea, skin rashes, diarrhea, insomnia, palpitations, and absent menstruation. These are signs that the diet should be moderated or stopped, and digestion kindled. It's always best to introduce an *āma*-cleansing diet or routine into your lifestyle slowly, under the guidance of an Ayurvedic practitioner. Those who are suffering from infectious illness, wasting disease, or emaciation; are under ten years or over seventy years; emotionally unstable; recovering from severe sickness; or otherwise very weak, should avoid cleansing and reducing therapies and instead focus on foods and treatments that rejuvenate and build.

What follows are a range of strategies to reduce *āma* accumulated in the food body. Some practices can be incorporated into the daily *dosha* diet, such as the first group here, based on the medicine of negation. Others are specifically cleansing. It is not necessary—or advised—to do everything at once. Begin with the medicine of negation, then add further cleansing approaches that suit your current health status, age, personal constitution, and the season. Begin slowly, and always observe the body for changes.

To help remove *āma* from the gut and tissues:

- *Stop taking in toxins*. Reduce or stop eating highly processed foods and ingredients, including junk foods and foods fried with or containing heat-extracted and hydrogenated oils. Whenever possible, avoid plant-based foods sprayed with agrochemicals, commercially farmed animals and their products, and foods manufactured using chemical methods and additives. Minimize the use of plastics as food wraps and storage vessels. Never heat foods in plastic containers. Avoid cheap and old nonstick pan coatings. Limit bottled and unfiltered water. Rethink the health and beauty products you use.

- *Avoid foods that easily increase āma*. While on a cleansing diet ideally avoid all dairy, meats, and animal products; all oily foods, fats, and oils; refined grains, sweeteners, and yeasted breads. Also avoid the nightshade vegetables (potato, tomato, capsicum, and eggplant). No cold beverages. No unsprouted nuts or seeds.

- *Avoid foods that cause signs of allergy or intolerance (often dairy and wheat)*. When we regularly take in aggravating foods, the body does its best to habituate, but can never be balanced. Sometimes the troublesome food(s) stimulate the adrenal glands to release stress-moderating hormones that actually help us feel better after eating. In this way the culprit's actions are masked, and problematic foods can become entrenched and even addictive. Food sensitivities can also trigger a mildly increased heart rate just after eating. The Coca Pulse Test monitors the heart rate after eating certain foods. At home, measure and compare the heart rate before eating and immediately after tasting or chewing suspect foods, even without swallowing. Other methods to detect food allergies include a five-day modified fast of simple foods such as *kitchari* (see recipe on page 202), followed by a test meal of the suspected food; a guided elimination diet; kinesiology or methods of energy testing; and skin-prick testing. To discontinue incompatible foods, it is often best to reduce quantities by one quarter each week over a four-week period.

- *Think twice about dietary supplements.* Marketeers convince us that food supplements are premium substances required to complete the diet and deliver energy, strength, good health, and beauty—yet manufacturers need not validate these claims. In reality, most food supplements are concentrated natural or man-made substances that are foreign to the body, and difficult to digest. The food body did not evolve with isolated, concentrated nutrients, removed from their living complex surroundings. The *agnis* may cope for a while, but the long-term effects are a gamble. If taking supplements, know and trust the formulation and source. For cleansing purposes, microalgae and young cereal grasses can be taken with water once or twice a day on an empty stomach—spirulina (one to two grams twice a day); wild blue-green algae (half to one gram twice a day); or wheat or barley grass shots or powder (two or more grams twice a day). Add citrus to pacify *vāta.*

Begin slowly, and remember that gentle is the best way. Further methods to reduce *āma* formation and cleanse the gut and tissues include:

- *Make dietary choices toward balancing your constitution.*
- *Use herbs to stoke the digestive fires and digest āma.* All efforts to eliminate *āma* hinge on the fiery force of *agni. Kapha* types can use pungent and bitter herbs such as dried ginger, black pepper, chili pepper, and cumin, or the Ayurvedic formula *trikatu; pitta* types can use bitter herbs such as barberry and turmeric, gentian, goldenseal (all good for *kapha,* too), or bitter *ghee,* cumin, coriander, fennel, fresh ginger, or the herbal mix known as *triphala; vāta* types can use dry or fresh ginger, cumin, fennel, cardamom, cinnamon, or dill.
- *Ensure the bowels are regular.* Ideally, we pass stool between one to three times a day, depending on *dosha,* diet, and lifestyle. Strategies to regulate the bowels include: balance the *dosha;* eat plenty of vegetables and drink ample warm water and supportive herbal teas; take two to four teaspoons of psyllium husk in the morning with plenty of warm water; take one to two teaspoons of *triphala* powder with warm water at night, just before bed; exercise regularly; and reduce mental and physical stress.

- *Choose raw and lightly cooked fruits and vegetables.* Fresh, raw foods such as salads, fresh herbs, and sprouts are high in air and ether, and inherently cooling, lightening, cleansing, nutritious, and contain helpful enzymes, but are more difficult to digest and assimilate than cooked vegetables and grains. In the general diet, *Āyurveda* encourages small amounts of raw foods—around 10 to 25 percent—served at room temperature, during the midday meal, in conjunction with cooked vegetables and grains. In warm, moist seasons more can be eaten, but *vāta* types should exercise caution. As part of a cleansing or reducing regime, robust *pitta* and *pitta-kapha* types can further increase raw foods, and often live comfortably on a raw diet for extended periods. In summer, as a cleansing strategy, over some days work your way up to between fifty to one hundred percent raw foods, maintain for a few days, then incrementally reduce to a mixed diet again.

- *Choose foods that help to neutralize and cleanse toxins.* From a Western perspective, nutrients including zinc, selenium, magnesium, iodine, sulfur, and silica play vital roles in bodily cleansing.

From an Ayurvedic standpoint, the tastes and qualities of foods indicate their actions. Enjoy bitter, pungent vegetables including kale, watercress, mustard greens, swiss chard, broccoli, Brussels sprouts, asparagus, fresh cilantro, daikon radish, turnips, garlic, onions, and shallots. For added effectiveness, mix bitter green vegetables with pungent red and orange varieties. Those who readily digest them can eat small to moderate amounts of well-prepared

Sprouts

Sprouted seeds, grains, and legumes produce enzymes that break down plant toxins, activate nutrients, and contain the intensely alive pigment, chlorophyll, equivalent to captured sunshine. Sprouted grains and grasses (wheat, barley) are cooling, hydrating, rejuvenating, and strongly cleansing. Sprouts stimulate the liver, oxygenate the blood, reduce heat and acidity, lower blood pressure, and can counteract the effects of low sunlight and artificial lighting. Sprout mung beans, fenugreek, and alfalfa. Juice wheat and barley grasses. In general, sprouts are ideal for *pitta*; assist *kapha* reduction (careful in wet, wintery environments); and for *vāta* are best lightly steamed or in summer.

mung beans, adzuki beans, black soybeans, tofu, brown rice, millet, rye, buckwheat, oats, barley, and corn (hold the genetic engineering). Unrefined sea and rock salts also have cleansing properties—best for *vāta* types, but should be minimized by *pitta* and *kapha* individuals.

- *Nurture the liver.* A healthy liver continuously filters the blood, identifies and deactivates toxins and would-be trespassers, digests and moves subtle substances, and creates a myriad of needed constituents. When the liver is clogged, stagnant, or overheated, all processes are hampered. To gently cleanse and nurture the liver, choose bitter substances such as salad greens, parsley, kale, watercress, alfalfa, dandelion greens, celery, rhubarb, aloe vera, saffron, gentian, goldenseal, and turmeric root. Seaweeds, spirulina, and wheat and barley grasses are also helpful, and avocado is a great liver rejuvenator. At meals, *pitta* types, and damp or overfed *kapha* types, and mixed *pitta-kapha* constitutions can do well to routinely commence meals with a salad of bitter greens. Bitter foods and herbs can be made more palatable by cooking them with sweet vegetables such as carrots, potato, or zucchini. *Vāta* types can steep mild bitter herbs to drink as tea. First thing in the morning, powdered bitters such as neem leaves (Azadirachta indica) or gentian (Gentiana lutea) and/or turmeric root (Curcuma longa) provide cleansing benefits. Take one-half teaspoon of each in warm water—but avoid if *vāta* is elevated. Other beneficial beverages include fresh ginger tea and chamomile tea. And fresh lemon juice or naturally fermented vinegar in tepid water—but *pitta* types beware. Plus, don't eat late at night, and ensure sufficient sleep.

- *Eat simple foods. Kitchari*, a wet meal of rice and dal, is *Āyurveda's* favorite light, cleansing meal. *Kitchari* can be used as a simple single meal, or food for the day, or longer. (See *Kitchari* recipe on page 202.) In general, combine fewer foods, such as lightly cooked green beans, celery, zucchini, and parsley; or eat a single vegetable or grain. Rice gruel is traditional. Soups are a good option. For oil, use small amounts of *ghee*.

- *Fast from food for a while.* Possibly the most effective way to reduce toxins in the system is to fast. In general,

Āyurveda supports a regular fast of one day every two weeks as part of a lifestyle routine. Controlled fasting allows the *agnis* to burn up toxins in the gut, liver, and deeper tissues. It also rests and rekindles the digestion, revitalizes the body and mind, enhances the sense of taste, loosens addictive behaviors, and improves our relationship with food. But fasting must be approached in a balanced way as needs and tolerance levels differ. *Vāta* types can fast on sweet fresh juice, milk or *lassi*, or broth for a meal, a day, or three. *Pitta* types can be challenged by hunger, but benefit from fresh pomegranate, apple, grape, or cucumber juice for up to three days. Heavy, robust *kapha* types can (and should) undertake the longest and most rigorous fasts. Bitter, astringent, or mildly sour juices or lemon water, ginger tea, or pure water can be taken for a few days or even a week. For all *dosha* types, *Āyurveda* suggests drinking a large glass of water first thing in the morning that has been stored overnight in a copper vessel. This helps to cleanse the stomach (whether you are fasting, or not). If at any time strength and energy levels unduly fall, a fast should be terminated.

A popular fasting approach today known as intermittent fasting fits each day's eating into a six-to eight-hour window. From an Ayurvedic perspective this could be termed rhythmic eating. The meal pattern may be an early breakfast and late lunch, or more commonly, a late breakfast or brunch (around 10:00 a.m., at the start of *pitta's* dominant hours) and early dinner (around 6:00 p.m., before the sun sets). This type of meal spacing allows sixteen hours to rest and rejuvenate the digestive fires. It is especially useful for *kapha* types and those needing to reduce excess *kapha dosha*. This style

Drink Fresh Juice

Āyurveda understands that juice extracted from fresh plants is high in *prāna*, readily assimilated, counteracts heat and acidity, and is inherently cleansing and healing. Juices are perfect if digestion is weak, or if few raw foods are eaten. Juice fresh, dark, green, leafy veggies along with other vegetables and fruits. Carrot and lemon juice make a good base (or organic apple for *pitta* types, or if you have a sweet tooth). Then, combine with two or three other ingredients. For extra digestibility and attributes, add fresh turmeric or ginger root or herbs such as mint or parsley. Drink juices during one- to three-day fast periods, or daily before or between meals.

of eating also has Yogic roots, and is common among spiritual seekers.

Additional strategies to help remove *āma* from the gut and tissues include:

- *Move the body.* Regular exercise helps to open up the body's physical and subtle channels to assist the flow of lymph, feces, sweat, and life-force *prāna*.
- *Combine Ayurvedic therapies* such as specific massage techniques, and heat and herbal treatments. Cleansing is amplified when dietary and lifestyle approaches occur in conjunction with specialized treatments under the guidance of an experienced practitioner. After a period of deep cleansing it is advised to undergo one or several cleansing, herbal enemas to remove mobilized toxins from the intestines. These can be done by practitioners—or self-administered.
- *Be gentle in body and mind.* Detoxing can cause temporary physical and mental unrest and discomfort as stored toxins and repressed emotions bubble to the surface. Be gentle with yourself as the system releases things that don't serve it. Before undergoing a period

of cleansing, contemplate the steps you'll take, tell the body your plans, and pledge to be attentive and supportive. Tell family and friends of your plans, and ask for their support. As your usual food intake reduces, employ other strategies to nourish the system such as deep breathing, loving thoughts, and mild practices of stretching, yoga postures and breath expansion, qigong, tai chi, and meditation that support physical and mental integration, clarity, relaxation, and balance. Continue these practices post-cleansing, as part of a daily routine, in conjunction with supportive diet and lifestyle.

Just Breathe

Breath charges the entire body with life-force; fortifies, cleanses, and relaxes the body and mind; keeps all substances flowing; balances the hormones; and reduces cravings for food, stimulants, and intoxicants. All *dosha* types benefit from *prānāyāma* practices, which include the Yogic breathing technique called *nādī shodana*, also known as channel cleansing or alternate nostril breathing. Learn *nādī shodana* from an experienced teacher, or have one check your technique. Practice five to ten minutes, once or twice a day while cleansing, and every day thereafter!

Sleep Sufficiently and Sweetly

Āyurveda considers sleep, along with food and sex, as the three pillars of life. Each of these three needs to be regulated. A set time for sleeping and adequate sleep allows organs to cleanse and regenerate—including the brain,[10] rests and balances the *dosha*, regulates the metabolism, reduces inflammatory processes, and supports nourishment, sexual prowess, knowledge, and happiness. In contrast, poor sleeping patterns upset the body's cleansing systems; imbalance the *dosha* (oversleeping aggravates *kapha*, and lack of sleep upsets *vāta*); strains the metabolism; drives hunger and indigestion; and creates *tamas*, low mood, and mental fog that reduce our ability to cope, and increase poor decisions and harmful tendencies.

From an Ayurvedic perspective, *vāta* types need most sleep and do best with eight to nine hours per night; *pitta* types are supported by seven to eight hours; and *kapha* individuals function best on six hours per night. Although they may fight it, ideally *kapha* types eat and sleep early, and rise before the sun. In general, the very young, very old, and the infirm need more sleep. In order to sleep better:

- Keep the digestive *agnis* balanced.
- Don't take caffeine and other stimulants late in the day.
- Eat a light, early evening meal at least two hours before bed.
- After sunset avoid bright household lighting; stay away from computer screens and devices. Instead enjoy calming lighting, sounds, and fragrances, and great works of fiction rather than fact-based information.
- Establish an evening practice of oil self-massage, warm bath, breathing exercises, and/or meditation.
- Before bed, oil the soles of the feet (then cover with woolen socks), and/or oil the ears and/or soak some cloth or cotton wool in oil and place between the eyebrows.
- In the northern hemisphere, don't sleep with the head pointing north. In the southern hemisphere, don't sleep with the head pointing south. The magnetic pull of the planet can place pressure on the brain and create restless sleep.
- Determine your ideal sleeping routine. Set an alarm to alert you when bedtime is approaching, and an alarm to wake up.

---

10   Using sedatives sedates the brain, which interferes with this function.

When undertaking a period of cleansing, consciously choose the best time, and learn along the way. A period of cleansing often constitutes an ideal step before initiating a *dosha* balancing diet and other therapeutic strategies. After cleansing, the system becomes lighter, more receptive, is reset, and can be deliberately rebuilt with balancing foods and habits. Cleansing and detoxification are healing therapies, but above and before this, *Āyurveda* sees them as preventative therapies to be used intermittently in conjunction with the lifetime *dosha*-balancing diet—such as a fortnightly day of fasting, plus one or two annual seasonal cleanses. And just as importantly, in order to avoid creating *āma* in the first place, is the practice of eating and living in balance with your unique mix of *dosha*. Let's take steps now.

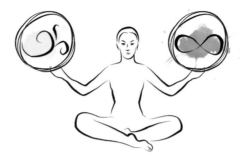

To balance vāta's dry, light, cold, rough qualities, choose moist, warm, soft, easy-to-digest foods.

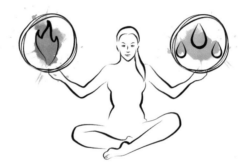

To balance pitta's moist, sharp, hot, light qualities, choose cool, soothing, and moderate.

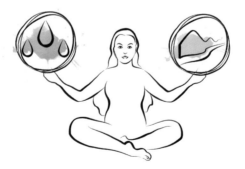

To balance kapha's wet, cool, heavy, dense qualities, choose dry, light, and warming.

CHAPTER 9

Living and Balancing Your Dosha (Constitution)

We are born with an innate mix of the five great elements. And over time, the foods and fluids we consume and the environments we live in add their elements and qualities to our own. A sour, warm, wet, sharp lemon; or the sweet, cold, heavy, cloudy, flowing qualities of milk introduce their elements and qualities into the food body. Recognizing the dominant elements and qualities in our physical body, and those dominant in the foods we eat bring an internal consistency and logic to nutritional thinking. To balance our constitution, we should limit foods high in qualities already dominant in our nature, and introduce more of the qualities that we lack. Foods are not *good* or *bad*. Rather, they are suitable or unsuitable according to the constitution of the eater; the time of day and season; and

qualities, quantities, and combinations of foods eaten.

A food that supports health in one person may incite disease in another. By recognizing our unique elemental makeup, examining the elements and qualities of foods, and the broader environment, we can make dietary choices that complement our *dosha* mix, rather than working in habit or ignorance against it.

After igniting the digestive fires and cleansing the body of *āma*, it's time to focus on the fundamentals of eating to balance the *dosha*. With a focus on practice, we examine eating according to taste and choosing foods for their elements and qualities; following a regular yet flexible

A question like: **is cheese good for me?**
 raises many considerations.
What is your constitution? Is there any *dosha*
 imbalance?
What kind of cheese? From what animal?
 What was that animal eating?
Is it made from homogenized or pasteurized
 milk?
How was it prepared or processed? Is it
 fermented or fresh?
What time of day do you want to eat
 cheese?
In what season?
How much will you eat?
What will you eat it with?
What time of life are you in?

meal pattern; and eating and living to cultivate the harmonious quality of *sattva*. A summary of eating and lifestyle guidelines for *vāta, pitta,* and *kapha* is also outlined below.

Eating for Taste

Āyurveda sees six primary tastes—sweet, sour, salty, pungent, bitter, and astringent—each created through a mix of the five great elements. Sweet/bland tastes are dominant in earth and water and have cool, moist, heavy, and building qualities. Sweet/bland tastes pacify *vāta* and *pitta dosha* but aggravate *kapha*. Sour tastes are dominated by fire and earth and have warm and mildly building qualities. Sour tastes pacify *vāta* but aggravate *pitta* and *kapha*. Salty tastes are dominant in fire and water and have warm and moist qualities. Salty tastes pacify *vāta* but aggravate *pitta* and *kapha*. Pungent tastes are dominant in fire and air and have hot, dry, light, and reducing qualities. Pungent tastes are beneficial for *kapha* but irritate *pitta* and *vāta*. Bitter tastes are dominant in air and ether and have cold, dry, light, and reducing qualities. Bitter tastes pacify *kapha* and *pitta dosha* but aggravate *vāta*. Astringent tastes are high in earth and air and have cool, dry, and heavy qualities. Astringent tastes pacify *kapha* and *pitta* but aggravate *vāta dosha*.

In all cases, optimal nutrition and balanced *dosha* are contingent on including all six tastes in the diet, adjusting the amounts according to constitution and season. We should emphasize the tastes that pacify our constitution, and include lesser amounts of the others. For everyone, foods sweet/bland in flavor should make up the majority of the diet—around 70 percent in *vāta* and *pitta* constitutions, and 55–60 percent in *kapha*. Examples of naturally sweet/bland foods include wheat, rice, barley, and most other whole grains; mung dal; most vegetables and fruits, especially pumpkin, zucchini, carrots, beetroot, potato; pineapple, melon, mango, bananas, sultanas and dates; seeds and nuts; fresh animal products; and most fats and oils.

Quell the Sweet Tooth

While the sweet/neutral taste should dominate, refined and artificially sweetened foods and beverages are not included in this list. As well as our biological calling for sweet, today refined sugars are added to almost all processed foods—breakfast cereals, biscuits, cakes, breads, milks, yogurts, desserts, salad dressings, soup mixes, canned foods, fast foods, bottled drinks, and alcohol—hiding behind labeling guises such as raw sugar, invert sugar, sucrose, glucose, fructose, high-fructose corn syrup, dextrose, maltose, lactose (and any other ingredients ending in -ose), maltodextrin, sugar syrup, corn syrup solids, all other syrups, fruit and fruit juice concentrate, molasses, maple syrup, and honey. Traditional *Āyurveda* had no such considerations. Within the current food environment, refined sugars, artificial sweeteners, and all man-made chemicals exist outside of nature. The digestive *agni* cannot fully digest these substances; they are imbalanced and unbalancing in nature. Unless labeled as *unrefined*, all sweeteners, including "organic" sugars are altered from their natural context. It is best to eat sweet/neutral whole foods.

Decreasing and ideally eliminating refined sweetness takes some vigilance, and our yearning for intensely sweet flavors is largely unhelpful. In *Āyurveda*, the herb *Gemnema sylvestra*, (commonly known as gurmar, or the *sugar destroyer*) temporarily blocks the sweet taste and is traditionally used to stop sugar cravings and help control blood sugar levels. Pure bitter herbs provide a similar effect. Bitter fenugreek seeds used in cooking or sprouted and eaten raw also help to regulate sugar metabolism, and are particularly balancing for *pitta* and *kapha*. If yearning for sugar, eating a sour food such as a citrus fruit, natural yogurt, or sauerkraut, can cut a craving. Micro algae such as chlorella (best for *vāta*), spirulina (good for *pitta or kapha*), or blue-green algae (best for *kapha*) taken before or between meals, or at the time of craving, can also quell the urge.

Sour Ferments

Today a number of sour foods dominate the Western diet, including breads, cheeses, yogurts, old foods, and alcohols. After sweet/bland tastes, the sour taste should be the next most common, especially for *vāta* types, where sour tastes might contribute around 20 percent, and *pitta* types the least, in the vicinity of 10 percent. Traditionally, many Indian cuisines have included sour, fermented foods at each meal, such as yogurt or *raita*, pickled fruits and vegetables, and chutneys. Other cultures have fermented grains to make breads; beans to soy, miso, and tempeh; cabbage to sauerkraut and kimchi; apples and other fruits to vinegar; and grains, fruits, and vegetables to alcohol.

In natural fermentation, bacteria, yeasts, and fungi spring to action, enlivening and partially digesting the food (and eventually bringing decay). Fermentation renders food more sour, acidic, and heating; and more flavorsome and digestible. Raw fermented foods provide digesting enzymes, feed the gut bacteria, support immunity, are a source of B12 for vegans, and are less perishable than the fresh ingredient.

Small regular servings of raw, naturally fermented foods support all constitutions. Enjoy one or two spoons of natural ferments before or during main meals. Produce your own yogurt, pickles, and breads as *wild* ferments, from naturally occurring bacteria, yeasts, and fungi.[16]

Unrefined Salts
To be sure, salts and the salty taste are an essential part of eating for health, but salts should only make up a small percentage of the total diet. Today, salt's bad rap is due to its refinement and overuse in food processing. As an ingredient,

salt is cheap, enhances shelf life and color, binds with water to increase weight (and therefore profitability), and enhances taste.

Refined salt is sodium chloride in a concentrated form, out of context with its complex source. In contrast, unrefined rock and sea salts contain complex mineral profiles. Unrefined sea salts possess a mineral balance similar to that of blood. Unrefined sea salt has a light grayish color, and Himalayan rock salt is slightly pink. Both come as crystals and powders.

When it comes to salty tastes, *vāta* types can indulge most, while *pitta* and *kapha* types are best to cultivate the love of fresh, natural foods with minimal addition of salt. All *dosha* types should use unrefined salt varieties in cooking and at the table, and avoid refined table salt and foods high in refined salts including processed foods, and ready-made meals and sauces.

The Lightening, Reducing Tastes
As well as their immediate effects on the metabolism, all tastes continue to influence the food body long after the meal is eaten. Following digestion in the gut and liver, some initial flavors take on different qualities and actions, known as *vipāka* or post-digestive taste. While sweet/bland tastes remain sweet and building, and sour

tastes remain sour, light, and heating, initially salty tastes become sweet and building, and pungent, bitter, and astringent tastes all become pungent and drying, lightening, and reducing in nature. Understanding the *vipāka* of foods tells us their longer-term building or lightening effect on the metabolism.

In their elemental mix, pungent, bitter, and astringent tastes all contain air and are dry and light immediately upon eating and also after digestion. For *vāta dosha*, these tastes introduce more air element, so should each make up only a small percentage of dietary intake. For *pitta* types, fiery pungent tastes should be minimized to a small percentage, but initially cooling bitter and astringent tastes can make up to 10 percent each, especially if longer-term lightening is needed. Bitter and astringent tastes generally cool *pitta* because their cold qualities and actions are stronger than the post-digestive pungency produced. In *kapha*-dominant individuals, pungent, bitter, and astringent tastes are the most balancing in the short—and long-term. Each can provide around 7 percent of daily intake. Using the post-digestive effect of foods helps to support long-term goals to lighten the food body when required.

As well as including all six tastes, it pays to support taste sensitivity. When taste perception is dull, the body can't properly prepare to receive inbound food, and satisfaction and digestion is affected. The extent to which we perceive food's flavors is evolutionary, biological, social, seasonal, relative, and also highly personal. The reception of taste also tends to diminish with age. The following are strategies to build taste awareness for enjoyment and good health.

- Learn how to combine foods and spices to create balanced, full-bodied meals. For example, in Indian vegetarian dishes, rich umami flavors that the tongue so enjoys are created by combining sweet, sour, salty, and spicy (pungent) tastes.
- At the meal table, pay attention to tastes, and practice distinguishing which flavors are present. Encourage children to eat a variety of foods; offer a new taste experience each week.
- Treat each taste as a doorway into a different reality. Observe the effects of different tastes on the physical and mental body.
- Don't mask or conceal the taste of medicinal herbs; allow them to be experienced as they enter the body.

- First thing in the morning, scrape the tongue to clean the taste buds and remove mucus and *āma*.
- In perceiving taste, smell is also important. If the nose is blocked, rinse the nasal cavity with lightly salted water using a technique known as *jala neti*. Complete the practice by rubbing a little oil in the nasal passages to prevent drying.
- Cleanse the palate and restore taste equilibrium by regularly eating bitter leaves and vegetables.
- Reduce or avoid alcohol, smoking, and drugs.

Eating Foods and Qualities

Ayurvedic wisdom relates to whole foods, wild-crafted by Mother Nature, or raised in and on fertile fields, processed suitably, gently and minimally. Enjoying these foods is the foundation of a healthy, balanced life. The approach of *Āyurveda* is inclusive. All-natural foods are recognized as potentially healing. For *Āyurveda*, the distinction of foods is in their elements and qualities, in particular heating and cooling, drying and moistening, and heavy (building) and light (reducing). Foods also contain the qualities of *sattva, rajas,* and *tamas,* which exert effects on the mind. Many natural foods are mild in their qualities. Some foods are relatively stronger in nature, a strength also relative to our constitution. When we eat foods high in qualities we already possess, habitual intake naturally leads to *dosha* imbalance. When we choose foods dominant in qualities opposite to our constitution or current imbalance, they promote *dosha* stability.

In Part I we looked at food groups and foods, and their elemental relationships with the *dosha* and the food body. In general, grains are mild and building for all *dosha*; vegetables are nutritive and cleansing; fruits are cooling, cleansing, and light; nuts, seeds, and oils are heating and heavy, as are most meats and animal products. When the daily and seasonal diet rotates through varieties of whole foods and taste combinations, qualities are tempered and mingled, and a wide range of foods can be enjoyed. Daily and seasonal variety ensures that all qualities are received, and none are overdone. Irrespective of constitution, *Āyurveda* encourages complementary food combinations, separating foods with contradictory qualities. Some basic principles of beneficial food combining (and separating) include:

- Enjoy fruits separately from other fruits and foods—thirty minutes before eating, or in between meals.

- Mix whole grains with other foods, especially vegetables.
- When combining grains and legumes, keep the emphasis on grains. Use a ratio of 2:1 or 3:1, or more.
- Mix dense, heavy foods, such as meat, with light, cooling green or watery vegetables. Acidic fruits such as lemons, limes, and tomatoes also mix well.

It's possible to antidote foods high in potentially unsuitable qualities with foods and preparation methods that introduce new qualities and reduce their effects—so we can eat a little, or a little more. Basic examples of antidoting include the following:

FOOD/QUALITY	ANTIDOTE
Sweet, heavy cheese; red meat	Black pepper; chili pepper
Warming eggs; fish	Fresh cilantro; parsley
Astringent legumes; cabbage	Garlic; ginger; cloves; turmeric; salt
Heavy nuts; seeds	Presoak or lightly dry-fry
Stimulating caffeine	Cardamom; nutmeg
Dry, frozen, or day-old refrigerated meals	Heat well, add extra digestive spices (e.g., ginger), and moisture (e.g., *ghee*)

Today, many people need more qualities of cooling, reducing, and cleansing, and less heating, building, and impurities. Of all food types, the natural qualities of animal products combined with modern factory farming techniques renders animal-based foods particularly problematic.

Mitigating Meat

In the short and long-term, the sweet-sour-salty-pungent combination of meat, fish, and poultry is heating, moistening, dense, and building which is useful to useful to build the body after illness and to pacify *vāta* (so long as they can digest it). For *pitta* types meats are innately unbalanced. For *kapha*-dominant individuals, the heating quality of meat is not such as issue (unless *pitta dosha* is also aggravated), but meat's moist, heavy, building nature renders *kapha* types and those with *kapha* dominance prone to congestion and weight gain.

Another way to characterize foods is by their effects on the mind. Diets high in meat feed *rajas* and *tamas* to the mind, while fresh, plant-based diets are generally higher in *sattva*, the universal quality that supports mental peace and harmonious *dosha*. Whole, plant-based foods also generally digest in less than half the time of meat, produce less *āma*, are cleansing and lightening, contain more complex tastes, are higher in vital life-force, and involve less violence than the killing of animals. However, for many people today, vegetables unaccompanied by a good cut of meat somehow lack substance and purpose. Meat is *the meal*. We feel satisfied by the rich heaviness of meat, are used to seeing it on our plate, and believe its removal deletes taste, bulk, and nutrition, leaving few worthy options. In most Western countries, meat-based diets have attained the momentum of many generations, and are literally built into our tissues. Until recently, eating meat was an act that required days of hunting, shepherding, tending, and killing creatures; or at the very least, was expensive to buy. But thanks to modern economics, science, industry, genetics, foods, and pharmaceuticals, meat is now cheap and readily available. Yet, its place in the diet can be questioned on health, environmental, and compassionate grounds.

In applying the medicine of negation, those with a weak digestion, *āma* conditions, imbalanced *pitta* or *kapha*, those looking to harmonize their mental state, and take in less toxins can benefit by eating less meat. Here are a few ideas how.

- Drop the mindset that meals must revolve around meat. Learn to cook satisfying alternatives. Select herbs, spices, and cooking methods to create rich flavors, and ingredients that provide chewiness and satisfying density and bulk. Explore garbanzos, beans, lentils, nuts, dense tofu, root vegetables, brown and sticky rice, whole grain pasta, and flat breads. Lightly steam your vegetables, and don't cook grains to pulp. Crown with a drizzle of cold-pressed oil and dusting of lemon juice or unrefined salt.

- Think about the animals you eat. Borders, time zones, miles, high-walled abattoirs, processing, packaging, and sauces physically and emotionally disconnect us from the animals we eat. Dining on flesh requires killing. But not doing the killing ourselves allows us to forget that living creatures must die so that we may live. Build compassion. Be grateful.

- Avoid factory farmed animals and their products, and the meat of animals that are emaciated, fatty, diseased, or poisoned.

- Only eat the flesh and products of animals who have been freshly killed and have eaten a diet that is natural for them in a natural environment. Support farming methods that consider the animal's nature, co-involve animals and

> **Digest the Meat You Eat**
>
> Pork, beef, mutton, dried meats, and meats prepared through dry, high-heat methods are very hard to digest, and flesh stagnating in damp, warm environments quickly turns acidic, feeds inflammation and bacteria, and encourages putrefaction. The most digestible, nourishing, and healing way to prepare meats is in broths, soups, and stews through slow, moist, low-heat cooking methods, including braising. Before cooking any meat, to complement taste and assist tissue breakdown and digestion, pre-marinade in pungent aromatic spices such as garlic, ginger, cardamom, clove, black pepper, cumin, chili, turmeric, or marjoram; and/or an acid medium of apple cider vinegar, lemon juice, or alcohol. Accompany meat dishes with dark green leafy vegetables or sulfur-containing vegetables such as onion, broccoli, or cabbage. A standard portion of meat should measure around half the size of the palm of your hand. Eat meat at lunch, when the digestive fires are strongest.

plants, are chemical-free, and preferably local to your area. Natural habitats are better for the animal, better for us, and better for the planet.

- In general, wild game, goat, chicken, and turkey (including thigh) is lighter, less heating, and easier to digest.

- Think about the fish you eat. Fish is warming, building, nutritious, and tasty but most seas are overfished and polluted, and freshwater farming is unsustainable. Rather than rely on fish for long-chain fats, obtain essential fatty acids from chia seeds, flaxseed, hemp seeds, mung beans, walnuts, chestnuts, Brussels sprouts, winter squash, dark green leafy vegetables, soy, barley, oats, rye, and microalgae such as spirulina and chlorella. If you eat fish, choose fish that have been raised in controlled, sustainable environments that have eaten a natural diet. Saltwater fish and seafoods (especially oysters) aggravate *kapha* and *pitta*.

- Eggs and natural dairy foods are ways to enjoy animal products that are nutritive and building, and involve less suffering.

- Choose your times. In colder climates, eating flesh can add needed warmth to the body that is harder to obtain through plant foods. Colder seasons also tend to produce a hotter digestion that can more readily process meat.

- Change your diet gradually. Begin by reducing your meat portion by one quarter, and continue to reduce by one quarter over weeks or months. A dramatic change away from meat can be shocking for the system and trigger food cravings. It takes the mind and the metabolism time to adjust to new tastes, new forms of nourishment, and increased lightness. Months, and often years, are required.

Dairy Decisions

Similar to meat, commercial dairy foods are hard to digest, and have become tainted by commercial farming and chemicals. Applying the medicine of negation, it's best for all *dosha* types and all ages to avoid dairy products that are homogenized, low fat, powdered, or "long-life." It may also be pertinent for children to avoid cow's milk for the first two years of life, especially if type 1 diabetes is known in the family. Nursing children should drink mother's breast milk in their first year of life.

In general, *Āyurveda* considers the best ways to enjoy dairy as fresh, full fat, chemical-free milk, fermented as yogurt, and as clarified butter, or *ghee*. But not in large amounts. Traditionally, milk and dairy foods were used more as a condiment to complement meals. Yogurt is best consumed churned with water, but not daily, or at night. An easy usage guide for *ghee* is one teaspoon per person in cooking, and for dry or emaciated *vāta* types or hot *pitta* individuals another half teaspoon on top of meals.

Assuming good quality milk is available, *vāta* types can benefit from its heavy, building qualities, especially when enjoyed warm, and prepared with mild pungent spices such as cinnamon, cardamom, fresh ginger, or nutmeg to assist its digestion. In moderation, the sour taste of fresh yogurt and dense salty qualities of cheese can also suit *vāta* types. For those with *pitta* constitution, the cooling quality of fresh milk and fresh cheeses such as cottage cheese and *paneer* can be useful. Those dominant in *kapha*, being heavy and cool by nature, are best to avoid most dairy. Goat's milk, which is lighter and more pungent, is a better choice.

Those with signs of milk or dairy intolerance, such as abdominal cramping, gas, and diarrhea tend to do better with fermented dairy products, or may do best to abstain from dairy for a time, or altogether—especially commercial varieties. Pasteurized milk can be better digested if brought to a quick boil then cooled. Almond and rice milks are good cow's milk substitutes that are easily homemade.

Drinking to *Dosha* Balance

Our daily fluid requirements vary according to constitution and *dosha* imbalance, diet, physical activity, living environment, work, travel, and season. In general, to stay cool and hydrated, individuals with *pitta* dominance require the most fluids—often upward of two liters (two quarts) per day, especially in warm climates. They benefit from tepid and room temperature water, plus sweet, bitter, or astringent teas. First thing in the morning (just after sunrise) drinking around half a liter (half a quart) of tepid water helps to hydrate and cool *pitta* constitution for the day. To assist water intake, a few drops of unrefined apple juice may help.

For those with *vata* constitution or *vata* imbalance, moderate to higher amounts of fluids are needed, especially in dry seasons and environments—one and a half to two liters (one and a half to two quarts) per day. Because *vata's* capacity to digest and assimilate water is less than *pitta* they may be best to drink small amounts more frequently. In particular, *vata* individuals benefit from warm to hot water, mineral water, warm spiced milk, broths, and spiced herbal teas. First thing in the morning (before sunrise) they can benefit from drinking up to one liter (one quart) of very warm water. A generous squeeze of fresh lemon or spoonful of apple cider vinegar is also cleansing and balancing.

Those with *kapha* constitution are already cool and moist, and generally require the least fluid, especially during wet seasons. First thing in the morning (before sunrise) they can benefit from drinking up to twelve ounces of warm water with lemon juice, or fresh ginger tea. During the day they might sip a little warm water and spiced or ginger tea. Spring water and boiled warm water are lighter options to help balance *kapha dosha*.

When it comes to tea and coffee, *vata* types and those with high *vata* are most vulnerable to their drying, stimulating effects; for *pitta*-dominant individuals they can be drying and heating; while in moderation, *kapha* types and those with *kapha* imbalance can benefit from these qualities. In general, tea and coffee are best consumed as a bitter digestive at the end of a meal. For those needing or wishing to cut down, grain beverages and bitter/astringent herbs are good post-meal options for all *dosha* types. Teas of alfalfa, dandelion, strawberry leaf, stinging nettles, hibiscus, chicory, and grain beverages are mildly digestive, cleansing, and antacid.

With regard to alcohol, these sour, pungent, sweet, bitter liquids can contribute digestive benefits, but can also readily disturb every *dosha*, and peace of mind. *Vata* types should stick to a little aged white or red wine, consumed after a warm, unctuous meal. *Pitta* types might enjoy a drop of aged red, or low alcohol beer while following a cooling regime, and after taking food that is moist and sweet. Those with *kapha* constitution can enjoy the odd nip of warming spirits such as brandy or rum or strong old wines, best taken after a light meal of grains mixed with black pepper. Always drink with awareness.

Being Regular Yet Flexible

Just as important as harmonizing the qualities of foods with those of our own constitution, *Āyurveda* recognizes that *how* and *when* you eat is also essential to balancing the *dosha*. Before hastily saying no to familiar foods, look first to your eating patterns, and say no to erratic and excessive habits that work against daily *dosha* cycles, tax digestion, and accrue *āma*. Replacing damaging habits with a suitably structured yet responsive meal pattern supports the digestive fires and all aspects of life. A few rules of thumb for all *dosha* types include:

- Eat your main meal in the middle of the day, while the digestive *agni* is strongest. (If you eat potentially aggravating foods, do it at lunch.)
- Eat only when hungry. When not hungry, digestion is not ready to accept food.
- Don't get too hungry. Avoid very delayed or random skipped meals.

- Ideally, eat your evening meal before sunset, or 7:00 p.m., or at least two hours before bedtime. And don't snack after dinner. Eating late taxes digestion, imbalances *kapha dosha*, and interferes with the body's nightly cleansing schedule.
- At home, don't eat out of saucepans, cookers, bags, containers, or hand-to-mouth off a platter. When serving yourself, or accepting from others, take your portion, and eat in one sitting. Don't take a small serving, planning to go back for seconds, or a pile of food, believing you will stop when full. Pack up leftovers immediately.
- Lose the mindset, *I can't waste it*. Only take what you need, but in the event that you have more than the stomach requires, keep it for the next meal, feed it to birds and animals, or compost it. No leftover food need be wasted. It is when we overeat that real waste occurs.
- Look out for feelings of deprivation. Most of us don't know genuine food insecurity, while a percentage of the world's population lacks access to adequate food. Is it right to feel deprived if we reduce our meal size, or forego a chocolate bar?

- Be aware that social situations ignite eating. The more people present, the more we tend to eat. In restaurants, think twice before ordering a larger portion that only costs a little more. You'll be served additional cheap ingredients, and you're still paying for food you don't need. If served too much, immediately send some food back. Minimize buffet restaurants that serve stale food, and overwhelm good sense. Try fresh, new alternatives and activities with family and friends that are less likely to incite old habits, and don't always center your activities around food.

Say No to Nibbles

A few decades back in a flash of insight, savvy food marketers recognized missed meals and the between-meal gap as profound business opportunities. From an energy boost for growing children, or sustenance for laboring adults, snacking morphed into the eating pattern of the modern generation. Today—car-bound, desk-bound, screen-bound—cheap, convenient snack foods are sandwiched between breakfast, lunch, and dinner; eaten in the absence of hunger; eaten in case we get hungry; gobbled by TV-light; savored by moonlight; or nibbled with drinks. Rather than food providing the medium

within which social events occur, snacks need no imperative or occasion. We're told it's normal to consume food any time of the day or night, alone or in company, on-the-move or standing, without reference to circumstance or hunger. While commercial snack foods generally come in smaller portions than main meals, their primary ingredients are notoriously refined sugars, fats, and salts, sprinkled liberally with preservatives and chemical additives. For convenience sake, we ignore the small amounts of poisons added to make foods inhospitable to bacteria, forgetting that the human gut hosts a colony of bacteria itself. Some snacks are labeled *healthy*, so we eat more of them.

From an Ayurvedic perspective, the snacking habit is a recipe for *dosha* imbalance. Whatever the food(s), constant nibbling weakens the digestive fires, which never have a chance to rest. Eating on top of a meal or before the previous meal is digested weakens and stalls the digestive process, creates mind-body fatigue and heaviness, and the likely production of *āma*. Plus, snackers frequently begin meals in a non-hungry state, alienated from natural rhythms of hunger and satiety. Amid social and environmental forces that fuel the snacking habit, *vāta* types enjoy the stimulation of snacks; *pitta* types try to dampen a nagging hunger; and *kapha* types can snack out of desire for comfort, or greed. To help counter a snacking habit:

- *Become aware of the times and situations that you snack, and want to snack.* Observe environmental/social/physical/mental/emotional aspects that trigger snacking—and workshop these motives directly.
- *Observe your snacking.* Turn the consumption of foods you feel attached or addicted to into an act of deep observance. If you eat junk food, pay attention to how it tastes, feels, smells, looks. Notice all ingredients. The fuller the experience the greater the satisfaction, but equally, paying close attention to the actual qualities of processed foods helps to loosen their grip on our tastes and desires.
- *Support the dosha and stabilize the digestive fires.* A balanced constitution and strong, steady digestion naturally harmonize appetite and hunger. When the constitution is balanced and digestion is strong, the body feels vital and nourished, and snacks lose their pull and appeal.
- *Prioritize a regular meal routine* so that you make fewer on-the-spot decisions that can create decision fatigue and feed the snacking impulse.
- *Don't buy snack foods when shopping.* And after twenty minutes of making multiple food decisions in the aisles, don't impulse buy at the counter.
- *If a snack must be had, the best choice is fresh fruit.* Fruit is light, hydrating, easily digested, quickly absorbed, cleansing, and ideally eaten alone. Enjoy one or two pieces.

In the process of restructuring meal and snacking patterns, quantities of unhelpful foods often need to be reduced before a food or habit can be changed. Downsizing unsupportive foods is best done slowly, cutting serving size by one quarter at a time. While in this process, ensure you still eat a sufficient overall quantity, adding as necessary familiar, enjoyable foods.

If an overall reduction in meal size is your goal, take three-quarters of your regular portion, and use small- to medium-sized bowls and plates that look fuller, rather than large vessels that we naturally wish to fill. You can monitor meal portions by using similar plates and vessels at each meal.

A daily meal pattern occurs within a *daily routine*, or *dinācharya*. A daily routine consists of lifestyle habits (waking, eating, acting, exercising, resting, sleeping) tailored to support *dosha* balance in conjunction with the environment you live in. In creating a regular yet flexible daily meal pattern, it's preferable first to work on structure and consistency before focusing on responsiveness and flexibility. With this in mind, let's look at basic eating and lifestyle guidelines for *vāta*, *pitta*, and *kapha*.

In the short-term, if two *doshas* are off balance, the most important *dosha* to work with is the one that first became imbalanced (most often *vāta dosha*). If unsure, work to pacify the *dosha* that is in greatest excess. If no imbalance exists, or as balance is restored, the primary and long-term focus of Ayurvedic nutrition is to maintain dietary and lifestyle patterns that support our natal constitution. This constitutes the lifetime basis for diet. Mixed *dosha* types should get to know both aspects of their constitution, and focus on working with the seasons and the *dosha* that is most vulnerable, and favoring overlapping or mutually beneficial tastes.

Guidelines for *Vāta Dosha*

Apply the Ayurvedic dictum *like increases like* to balance *vāta's* dry, light, cold, rough qualities. Avoid or eat sparingly the following:

- Spicy, bitter, and astringent-tasting foods

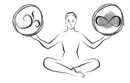

- Dry foods such as popcorn, crackers, chips, dry cereals, biscuits; frozen and dehydrated foods; un-soaked nuts and dried fruit
- Cold foods and drinks from the fridge or containing ice
- Frozen foods including processed meals and fresh meals that have been frozen
- Gas-forming foods such as cabbage, dried beans, and peanuts
- Raw foods, especially in cold seasons (always use oily/creamy dressings)
- Stimulating substances such as black tea, coffee, and refined sugar

Apply the Ayurvedic dictum *opposites reduce* to support *vāta dosha* and choose a regular meal pattern of moist, warm, soft, easy-to-digest foods. Emphasize:

- Local, seasonal foods that are naturally sweet/bland, sour, and salty in taste
- Moist, unctuous, freshly cooked foods such as whole grain porridges, root vegetables, soups, stews, *kitchari*, gravies, omelets, and custards

- Fresh, pre-soaked or lightly roasted seeds and nuts such as almonds, sunflower seeds, sesame seeds, walnuts, pine nuts; and nut milks and pastes
- Fresh, organic milk from cows, goats, almonds, coconut, and rice (Warm and add spices; sweeten if desired)
- Natural yogurt and sweet/salt/spiced *lassi*
- *Ghee* , or oils of sesame, peanut (ground nut) avocado, coconut, or olive in cooking, or over fresh and cooked dishes
- Unrefined cane sugars and syrups, jaggery, molasses, dates, a little honey
- Warming, digestive spices such as garlic, cardamom, cinnamon, nutmeg, basil, cloves, coriander, cumin, turmeric, asafoetida, fenugreek, and rock salt.
- Pickled vegetables and sauerkraut
- Warm fluids including water; lemon water; milk; broths; herbal teas of cardamom, cinnamon, clove, ginger, orange, lemon, mint, rosemary, anise, and chamomile
- Fresh fruit/vegetable juices

Daily Menu Planning for *Vāta Dosha*

Breakfast (light to medium in size)

Cooked or fresh seasonal fruit or fruit smoothie: 1 serving
Ingredients: Apricots, mangoes, berries, cherries, pears, grapes, banana, kiwi, citrus, papaya, pineapple, peach, avocado. Eat first.

Cooked whole grain cereal: 1 serving
Ingredients: Oats, wheat, rice, amaranth, quinoa, and milk. If desired, add *ghee*; unrefined sweetener; pre-soaked or ground-up dried fruits, nuts, or seeds

Herbal tea: 1 cup

Lunch (medium in size; the main meal)

Unctuous, cooked, seasonal vegetables: 1 serving
Ingredients: Carrot, beetroot, sweet potato, pumpkin, parsnip, turnip, asparagus, radish, mustard/turnip greens, snow peas, green beans, okra, onions, garlic. Sauces; warming spices (such as ginger, turmeric, cumin, nutmeg, thyme, basil, rosemary, dill); *ghee*; oil; lemon or lime

Well-prepared whole grains: 1 serving
Ingredients: Rice (basmati, brown, red), wheat, quinoa, couscous, spelt as meal base or in soups, pastas, stews. Millet and rye occasionally.

Green salad with vinegar/lemon, oil: ½–1 serving (optional)

Pulses; dairy; eggs; meat; seeds: 1 serving, 2–4 times a week
Ingredients: Split mung beans, red lentils, adzuki beans, tofu; churned yogurt (*lassi*); cheese; cream; scrambled egg(s)/omelet; fish; chicken; turkey, venison; goat; nut or seed paste

Herbal tea: 1 cup

Snack (only if genuinely hungry)

1 serving
Ingredients: Fresh fruit; pre-soaked dried fruit or nuts; un-yeasted bread with avocado or *ghee/*butter and/or sweetener; natural yogurt, *lassi*, or cottage cheese with sweetener or warming spices; a small handful of fresh sunflower seeds or toasted pumpkin seeds

Dinner (light to medium in size)

Whole grains: 1 serving

Spiced vegetables: 1 serving

Pulses; dairy; eggs; meat; seeds: ½–1 serving, 2–3 times a week

Herbal tea: 1 cup

Herbal Therapies for Vāta Dosha

A common digestive formula to support *vāta's* weak, irregular digestion is equal amounts of powdered seeds of cardamom, cumin, and fennel. Classically, small amounts of asafoetida (*hing*) are also mixed in. Take one teaspoon with warm water before meals.

Rejuvenating herbs that support *vāta dosha* include *amalaki* (Phyllanthus emblica), *ashwagandha* (Withania somnifera), *bala* (Sida cordifolia), garlic, licorice root (Glycyrrhiza glabra), *shatavari* (Asparagus racemosus), *tulsi* (Ocimum tenuiflorum), *vidari* (Pueraria tuberosa), and *triphala* (a mix of equal parts of three dried, powdered fruits—*amalaki* (Emblica officinalis), *bibhitaki* (Terminalia bellirica), and *haritaki* (Terminalia chebula).

Basics of Lifestyle for Vāta Dosha

- Three regular meals within a regular daily routine.
- Sleep early (ideally by 10:00 p.m.), and for eight to nine hours. Sleep on the left side to stimulate warming solar energies.
- Rise at least thirty minutes before dawn.
- Open the bowels daily.
- Stay warm; avoid cold, windy conditions.
- Spend time in tranquil, protected environments.
- Regularly massage the body with warm sesame, peanut (ground nut), or almond oil, then dress warmly and in twenty minutes take a warm shower, or if evening, go to bed.
- Breathe calmly and deeply. Prioritize five to ten minutes of alternate nostril breathing (*nādī shodana*) morning and evening.
- Enjoy gentle yoga postures that stimulate the pelvic area, involve balance, and cultivate stillness, grace, and body and breath awareness; and walks, especially in the early morning. Other suitable activities may include hiking, horseback riding, golf, swimming, sailing, canoeing, cycling, flowing dance, ballet, non-violent aikido, tai chi, qigong, Pilates, stretching, badminton, ping pong, bowling, baseball, cricket, light treadmill or stair-stepping, low impact aerobics, light gym workouts, and light weight training.

Guidelines for *Pitta Dosha*

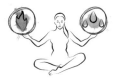

Apply the Ayurvedic dictum *like increases like* to balance *pitta's* moist, sharp, hot, light qualities. Avoid or eat sparingly the following:

- Pungent (spicy), sour, and salty-tasting foods
- Refined oils and sugars, fried foods, red meat, sea fish, hard cheese, caffeine, alcohol
- Steaming hot foods and drinks

Apply the Ayurvedic dictum *opposites reduce* to manage *pitta dosha*. Think cool, soothing, and moderate. Emphasize:

- Sweet/bland, bitter, and astringent tastes
- Salad greens and vegetables
- Sweet seasonal fruits
- Well-prepared whole grains and cereals, beans, and lentils
- Fresh milks from cows, goats, almonds, coconut, rice; cottage cheese; sweet *lassi*
- Small amounts of *ghee* (bitter *"tikta" ghee* is ideal), or oils of sunflower, olive, or coconut in cooking, or over fresh and cooked dishes. Sprinkle coconut or sunflower seeds.

- Unrefined sugar, date or palm sugar, barley malt, maple syrup, apple purée, dates, honey (if *pitta* is balanced)
- Sweet, neutral spices in moderation—fennel, coriander, cardamom, cinnamon, turmeric, cumin, mint, parsley, rock salt
- Room temperature water; sweet/bitter/astringent herbal teas such as barley, fennel, chamomile, chicory, dandelion, nettle, alfalfa, saffron, rose, mint, hibiscus, jasmine, lemongrass, lavender, raspberry, red clover; fresh juices

Daily Menu Planning for *Pitta Dosha*

Breakfast (medium to large in size)

Sweet fruit/juice/fruit smoothie:
1–2 servings
Ingredients: Grapes, pomegranate, peach, nectarine, apricot, plums, pears, apple, figs, cherries, berries, orange, pineapple, melon, mango. Eat first.

Cooked or pre-soaked whole grain cereal:
1–2 servings
Ingredients: Cracked or rolled wheat, oats, kamut, spelt, granola, barley, and milk or water. If desired, add unrefined sweetener; dried fruits

Herbal tea: 1 cup

Lunch (medium to large; the main meal)

Bitter green salad: 1 serving
Ingredients: Leaves, herbs, cucumber, sprouts, celery. Lime dressing and/or oil. Eat first.

Cooked whole grains: 1–2 servings
Ingredients: Barley, rice (basmati, brown, red, wild), oats, wheat, couscous, amaranth, unleavened bread

Lightly cooked seasonal vegetables: 1–2 servings
Ingredients: Green beans, cabbage, broccoli, Brussels sprouts, cauliflower, cucumber, celery, zucchini, leafy greens, okra, peas, asparagus, squash, sweet corn, mushrooms, potato, carrots, cooked white onions. Mild spices or fresh herbs such as cilantro or parsley on top

Pulses; dairy; eggs; meat: 1 serving, 4–6 times a week
Ingredients: Mung, adzuki, lima, kidney beans; garbanzos; split peas; black lentils; soy beans, tofu, tempeh; dairy; egg whites; chicken, turkey, venison; freshwater fish

Herbal tea: 1 cup

Snack

Preferably not. Or choose sweet fruit, dates, cranberries, sunflower or pumpkin seeds, fresh or dried coconut, fresh milk or *lassi*

Dinner (light to medium)

Green salad: 1 serving

Whole grains: 1–2 servings

Seasonal vegetables: 1–2 servings

Pulses; dairy; eggs; meat: 1 serving, 2–3 times a week

Herbal tea: 1 cup

Herbal Therapies for Pitta Dosha

A common digestive formula to cool *pitta's* hot *agni* is equal amounts of powdered seeds of fennel, coriander, and cumin. Take one teaspoon with warm water with meals. Try also one-half teaspoon of bitter *ghee* in warm water in the morning.

Rejuvenating herbs that support *pitta dosha* include *amalaki* (Emblica officinalis), aloe vera (Aloe barbadensis), *gotu kola* (Centella asiatica), licorice root (Glycyrriza glabra), *triphala*, *shatavari* (Asparagus racemosus), pomegranate juice.

Basics of Lifestyle for Pitta Dosha

- Three regular, satisfying meals.
- Sleep early (ideally by 10:00 p.m.), and for seven to eight hours. Sleep on the right side to stimulate cooling lunar energies.
- Rise at least forty-five minutes before dawn.
- Void the bowels first thing every morning.
- Spend time in relaxed, non-competitive environments.
- Keep cool. Stay out of the sun; avoid excess steam and humidity; get plenty of fresh air. After eating, place wet fingers over the eyes to temper the rise in *pitta*.
- Regularly massage the body in the morning or afternoon, or when you feel hot or dry, with cooling oils such as coconut, sunflower, or olive. Wait twenty minutes, then take a warm shower, or if evening, go to bed.
- Breathe calmly and deeply. Prioritize five to ten minutes of alternate nostril breathing (*nādī shodana*) morning and evening.
- Enjoy regular exercise during cooler hours. Practice yoga postures that stimulate the navel area, are not overly detailed or technical, and turn the focus inward. Consider team sports that emphasize cooperation and downplay aggression such as volleyball, hockey, basketball, and netball. Try self-competing pursuits that work toward realistic goals such as cycling, golf, hiking, mountain biking, surfing, kayaking, rowing, sailing, water skiing, wind surfing, water polo, swimming in open-air pools, diving, archery, martial arts, racquet sports, ball sports, snow sports.

Guidelines for *Kapha Dosha*

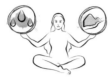

Apply the Ayurvedic dictum *like increases like* to balance *kapha's* wet, cool, heavy, dense qualities. Avoid or eat sparingly:

- Sweet/bland, sour, and salty tastes, including refined sugars and salts
- Refined oils, hard fats, fried foods
- Animal-based foods, especially dairy, saltwater fish, and fatty meats
- Nuts and seeds
- Cold foods and cold and iced drinks
- Sweet, heavy fruits such as banana, mango, avocado, coconut, figs, and dates
- Snacks

Apply the Ayurvedic dictum *opposites reduce* to manage *kapha dosha*. Think dry, light, and warming. Emphasize:

- Pungent/spicy, bitter, and astringent tastes
- Green salads and seasonal vegetables
- Warm, drying whole grains and light foods such as crackers and roasted/ puffed grains
- Digestible beans and legumes
- Astringent, mildly sour, or dried fruits
- Drizzle *ghee*, or mustard, sunflower, or corn oil. Sprinkle pumpkin or sunflower seeds
- Honey (but don't cook or overheat it). Unrefined stevia leaf
- Warming, lightening spices. Garlic, ginger, chili pepper, mustard, black and white pepper, turmeric, cardamom, cloves, cinnamon, cumin, fenugreek, basil
- Warm water; bitter/astringent/spicy herbal teas such as fresh ginger, alfalfa, dandelion, black pepper. A little honey in warm water, plus lemon juice and a pinch of black pepper, if desired. Celery and green vegetable juices. If not congested, small amounts of goat's milk or fresh buttermilk

Daily Menu Planning for *Kapha Dosha*

Breakfast (eat only if hungry)

Sour or astringent fruit: 1 serving

Ingredients: Grapefruit, passionfruit, pomegranate, young stone fruit, cranberries, apple, currents

Spicy tea: 1 cup

Lunch (main meal)

Bitter green salad: 1 serving
Ingredients: Leaves, herbs, sprouts, celery.
Apple cider/balsamic vinegar; lime; lemon. Eat
first.

**Steamed/stir-fried/roasted seasonal
vegetables: 2 servings**
Ingredients: Garlic, onions, leeks, scallions,
cabbage, celery, beetroot, beet/mustard/radish
greens, kohlrabi, asparagus, artichokes, capsicum,
green beans, salad greens, spinach, turnips,
radishes, carrots. Season with warming spices.

Whole grains: ½ –1 serving
Ingredients: Buckwheat, millet, barley, brown or
red rice (especially brown basmati), corn, rye,
amaranth, quinoa, sorghum, toasted flat bread.
Before cooking, dry-roast grains in a heavy pan
to lighten and increase digestibility.

Pulses: 1 serving, 2 times a week
Ingredients: Mung, adzuki, pinto, lima beans; lentils;
garbanzos; split peas; tofu/tempeh (cautiously)

**Animal products: 1 serving, 1 -2 times a week
(optional)**
Ingredients: Chicken; goat; venison; freshwater
fish; egg(s)

Herbal tea (if thirsty): 1 cup

Snack

Say, no thanks! Snacking dampens and burdens
Kapha's slow digestion

Dinner (warm and light)

Steamed or roasted vegetables: 1–2 servings

Whole grains: ½ –1 serving

Pulses: ½ –1 serving

Herbal tea (if thirsty): 1 cup

Herbal Therapies for Kapha Dosha

A digestive formula to support *kapha's* slow
digestion is equal amounts of powdered ginger
root, black pepper, fenugreek, and cumin. Take
one teaspoon with warm water after meals.

Rejuvenating herbs that support *kapha dosha*
include *ashwagandha* (Withania somnifera),
black pepper (Piper nigrum), garlic, *guggulu*
(Commiphora wightii), *gokshura* (Tribulus ter-
restris), myrrh (Commiphora myrrha), *pippali*
(Piper longum), *triphala*, *tulsi* (Ocimum tenuiflorum), and *shilajit* (Asphaltum).

Basics of Lifestyle for Kapha Dosha

- Two meals per day eaten between 10:00 a.m. and 6:00 p.m. is ideal for most *kapha* types.
- Fast from meals and solid foods at regular intervals.
- Sleep by 11:00 p.m., for six hours. Sleep on the left side to stimulate warming solar energies.
- Rise at least ninety minutes before dawn. No daytime naps.[11]
- Void the bowels first thing every morning.
- Spend time in warm, dry, secure environments; avoid cold, damp conditions.
- Before showering, rub the skin with a mitt or loofah of rough natural fibers in the direction of the torso to stimulate circulation and lymphatic drainage. In cold, dry seasons consider a light oil massage (morning or midday, if possible) with oils such as corn, almond, olive, or sesame. Wait twenty minutes, then take a warm shower.
- Breathe calmly and deeply. Prioritize five to ten minutes of alternate nostril breathing (*nādī shodana*) morning and evening.
- Enjoy daily physical activity. Practice strong forms of yoga such as *ashtanga* and series of postures that bring energy to the chest and head, and increase the heart rate and depth of breathing. Engage in lively, varied physical pursuits such as vigorous walking, hiking, jogging, cycling, stair-stepping, rowing, competitive swimming, water polo, cross-country skiing, ice hockey, skating, aerobics, gymnastics, martial arts, handball, lacrosse, tennis, racquet ball, soccer, rugby, volleyball, fencing, shot put. Build movement into every hour of the day.

Dual-Type Constitutions

Dual *dosha* types should eat to pacify an aggravated side of their constitution, and always consider the seasons. In spring and summer, those with *pitta-vāta* constitution can eat to pacify *pitta*, and in fall and winter pacify *vāta*. In general, chosen flavors should emphasize sweet, and minimize pungent. *Pitta-kapha* types can focus on pacifying *pitta* from late spring to early fall, then support *kapha* through to early spring. Bitter and astringent tastes are especially harmonizing, while sour and salty tastes shuld be enjoyed with care. In late winter and spring, *kapha-vāta* constitution can eat to pacify *kapha*, and in fall and early winter pay more attention to *vāta*. In summer choose according to whether the elements of water or air

---

11   Day-time sleep aggravates *kapha dosha*, digestion, circulation, and breathing, but can benefit aggravated *vāta* types, and those fasting or convalescing. In summer, a short daytime nap can help cool *pitta* and calm *vāta* within all constitutions.

dominate alongside heat. To add heat to this cold constitution, favor the warming tastes of sour, salty, and pungent. Enjoy more cooling tastes in summer, and astringent and bitter in spring.

Practicing *Sattva*

Of the three complementary forces of Mother Nature—*sattva*, *rajas*, and *tamas*—*sattva* is the equilibrium or middle ground that brings illumination, harmony, and balance to the process of creation. A mind dominated by *sattva* is intelligent, clear, peaceful, perceptive, intuitive, flexible, and responsive to changing events. In the body, *sattva* supports all three *dosha*, and physical and mental rejuvenation. Indian traditions understand that *sattva* also promotes spiritual ascendance. To bring joy, harmony, intelligence, and flexibility to our daily meal pattern and choices, *sattva* is an ideal support.

In general, the *sattvic* quality is high in foods that are grown gently in harmony with Mother Nature, on rich soils, and are naturally ripened, fresh, and freshly prepared. These foods are high in life-force *prāna*, naturally sweet, mild, and easy to digest. In a *sattvic* diet, some foods can be eaten raw, but most meals are lightly cooked (preferably by someone who is high in *sattva*), and eaten in moderation. To increase *sattva*, first apply the medicine of negation, and limit or avoid foods that are excessively *rajasic* or *tamasic* in nature.

> ### *Rajasic* Foods
>
> Foods that are *rajasic* in nature include pungent foods, especially garlic, onions, chili pepper, asafoetida (*hing*), and intense spices; strong sweet, sour, or salty flavors, including fermented foods, and meats; stimulants including caffeine; foods that cause flatulence such as dried and improperly prepared beans; cold, dry, rough foods such as those straight from fridge, and dry crackers, popcorn, and nuts. Alcohol and most other drugs are initially *rajasic* then become strongly *tamasic*. All stimulants (including garlic, onions, and chili pepper), initially stimulate the nervous system, before depleting and desensitizing it. *Rajasic* foods must be fresh and freshly prepared or else they become *tamasic*. Under-eating is *rajasic* in nature.

> ### *Tamasic* Foods
>
> Foods that are *tamasic* in nature include those that are old, stale, contaminated, and decaying, such as those engineered for a long shelf life; foods overly processed or overcooked; commercial meats, fish, eggs, and dairy; products that contain chemical additives and pollutants; foods that make us dull or sleepy; alcohol and drugs. Too many bitter and astringent foods can also induce *tamas*. All over-eating is *tamasic*.

Foods that are dominant in *sattva* include:

- Freshly cooked whole grains, especially basmati rice and cracked wheat
- Freshly cooked vegetables, especially root vegetables and squash
- Mung beans (whole or split, cooked or sprouted)
- Sweet seasonal fruits; a little lemon and lime; dried fruits
- Fresh seeds and nuts, especially pine nuts, and pre-soaked, peeled almonds
- Fresh milk from happy, healthy cows
- Sweet or mildly spiced *lassi*
- *Ghee* (clarified butter)
- Unrefined sweetener, especially honey (drink in warm water)
- Mild spices—fennel, cumin, coriander, turmeric, cinnamon, cardamom, black pepper, fresh ginger, basil, mint
- Pure water and ginger tea

Throughout life, the qualities of *sattva*, *rajas*, and *tamas* enter us through the foods we eat, and also through the five sense organs from our surroundings and the company we keep. Additional ways to cultivate *sattva* therefore include consciously choosing conditions that incorporate peace, love, happiness, truth, beauty, and coherence. Surround yourself with people who practice kindness, compassion, honesty, humility, service, gratitude, and forgiveness, and promote social environments that support *sattvic* ideals. Work on seeing life more clearly, without filters or bias. Allow life to unfold at a natural pace. Sit with decisions rather than habitually diving in. Open and express what's in your heart. Make food and lifestyle choices based on humanitarian and compassionate grounds. Choose minimalism and simplicity over materialism and complexity.

Sattva lives in natural habitats. Consciously be in tune with Mother Nature. Respond to her seasons and cycles. Spend time in expansive environments such as fields, mountains, forests, oceans, and sweeping terrains. The food body is physically constrained, but the fields of the four subtle bodies can expand indefinitely. Despite the matter-of-factness of modern science, look in awe at the profound arrangement of the universe. Ponder the vastness and be humbled and transformed by your diminutive perspective. Nurture your reciprocal relationship. Support vibrant oceans and forests. Plant trees and perennial vegetation; grow veggies, herbs, and flowers.

As well as directing ourselves towards *sattvic* activities, *sattva* can be cultivated by selectively withdrawing the senses from excessive and unsettling stimulation. Instead of overburdening the eyes, ears, tongue, nose, and touch, allot time, or in everyday life, consciously withdraw one or more of the senses, and rest. Turn away from screens, don't listen to small talk, avoid speaking needlessly, and rest quietly within. Practicing sensory withdrawal reduces the *rajas* and *tamas* we bring in, and rejuvenates the senses. The practice of sense withdrawal is the fifth limb of the eight limbs of yoga, followed by concentration, and meditation. A goal of all of these activities is to direct the mind and senses intelligently, to simplify thinking, and create gaps in the flow of thought. Many methods of sense withdrawal, concentration, and meditation exist and can be tailored to individual *dosha* type and tendencies. Airy *vāta* types who can't sit still might begin with mindful activity such as walking, qigong, tai chi, or yoga postures, followed by repetition of a *mantra*, or a visualization. Fiery *pitta* types who consider meditation an unproductive use of time and spend it analyzing and planning, can put their natural discipline to organized rituals, cooling *prānāyāma*, a *mantra*, or guided meditation. Earthy *kapha* types can invigorate and direct a dull mind with meditative walking or dance, dynamic yoga postures and *prānāyāma*, and martial arts. Devotional practices such as meditating upon a *guru* (enlightened spiritual master) or deity (bhakti yoga) may also suit. Choose whatever appeals to you.

To change the content of the mind does require effort, but it need not be overly difficult or protracted. To begin, become more aware of your thoughts and actions. And do something every day with a *sattvic* goal. One thing done consciously far outweighs a number of things done chaotically or unconsciously.

A Tree Is a *Sattvic* Lesson in Life

While Hindu philosophy has associated trees with *tamas* due to their non-moving (rooted) nature, this also provides trees with great stability—a quality that humans can aspire to. But more than *tamas*, in trees *sattva* is the quality that reigns. In life, trees live and grow according to their intelligent, feeling nature, responding to hot and cold, dryness and moisture, dark and light. A tree represents serenity, patience, and resilience. As trees spread out and face the sun, winds, and rain, they live and die in the service of others. In the atmosphere, trees purify the vital life-force *prāna*, remove hazardous carbon dioxide, and harness the sun. With these inputs they manufacture life-sustaining oxygen and sugars. Trees hold humidity in the atmosphere; control soil moisture and erosion; provide shade and exquisite fruits; offer shelter and fodder to animals; and produce healing remedies of barks, roots, resins, branches, flowers, fruits, and leaves. Trees provide fragrance and beauty; they reach from Earth toward heaven and support places for mediation and spiritual insight. Trees offer materials for clothing and tools; wood for fuel, transport, and construction; and a means of economic wealth. Even in death, trees bequeath their physical remains to throngs of microbes who create new fertile soil. For human-kind, trees are protectors of natural balance, and stabilize and nourish our existence on Earth—insofar as we nurture and protect them ourselves. Plants can live very well without humans, but humans cannot live without plants.

Vrikshāyurveda, an arm of *Āyurveda* dedicated to the health of plants, understands that the planting of trees provides a basis for fulfilling the four goals of Hindu life: duty, material wel-fare, pleasure, and spiritual emancipation.[17] In the light of the current global ecological crisis, saving and planting trees is perhaps our best and most tangible strategy. The great Indian Buddhist emperor, Ashoka, encouraged all citi-zens to plant and look after a minimum of five trees in their lifetime—one medicinal tree, one fruiting tree, one for firewood, one for hardwood, and one tree for flowers. This sounds like a good start. Plant trees indigenous to your area.

A Body-Ful Meditation

Sit in a comfortable position with your back straight. If this is not possible, you can lie down.

Close your eyes, and breathe in deeply through the nose, bringing the air all the way into the belly. Let the belly rise and hold the breath momentarily. As you exhale let the belly fall, and breathe out all tension and thoughts. Repeat three times.

Now, focus your awareness on the *food body*. Bring the mind into the physical body, and let it roam around. Feel into every limb, space, and channel. Experience the heaviness and solidity of the food body. Feel it as a whole.

When you are ready, shift your attention to the *vital* or *breath body*. This subtle sheath perme-ates the food body and extends beyond. See and feel the *prānic* sheath flowing smoothly and effi-ciently, circulating vital life-force throughout every aspect of being. Now, bring your aware-ness to the *mental body*. Imagine this energy field permeating and extending beyond what you know as the body. Rather than be lost in thought, experience the mental field surround-ing and supporting you peacefully.

Next, bring your awareness to the *wisdom body*. This even-more-subtle sheath suffuses the men-tal, vital, and physical sheaths, and operates beyond their processes. Experience the wis-dom body, merged with the field of universal intelligence. The source of intuition and deep knowing.

Now, extend your awareness to the *bliss* or *causal body*. At home in the subtle heart center, experience the infinitely subtle bliss sheath diffusing in all directions, enveloping and resonating throughout and beyond your entire being.

After experiencing the bliss body, envisage and experience all five bodies coexisting in balance and harmony. Remain with this attitude for some time. Move your attention back through each body. Spend as much time in awareness of each body as you like. Or just focus on the body as a whole.

Then, bring your consciousness to the food body. Experience your deep connection with Mother Earth, and Mother Nature.

Finally, do whatever else you feel would complete this meditation. Then, smile (if you aren't already), and slowly open your eyes.

CHAPTER 10

Embodied Eating and Living

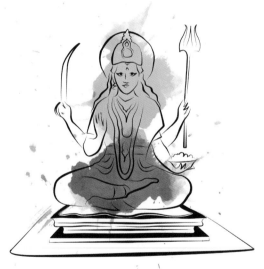

Annapurna

The goddess of food and nourishment

Āyurveda positions food as a gift from the universe and sacrifice to the digestive fires that should involve gratitude, awareness, and reverence. In moving toward this consciousness, embodied eating deepens our food, body, worldly, and cosmic relations through the fundamental actions of paying attention to where our food comes from; handling and eating it with all senses; expressing gratitude and respect, if not reverence for food. And consciously observing the entire experience. Embodied eaters give themselves space to monitor internal and external events from within a structured meal pattern. Through their attention, embodied eaters become grateful, receptive, and responsive. By deepening important relationships they elevate the eating experience. This chapter covers a vital aspect of Ayurvedic nutrition, coined here as *embodied eating*. Read on to become a more embodied, attentive, receptive, responsive eater. Topics of focus include hunger, cravings, satiation, bodily wastes, the five elements and senses, mental constructs, feelings, and intuition. We delve into conscious cookery, and build true appreciation of food. As we get underway, let's commence by truly paying attention.

Attention

In an old Zen story, a student asks his master to "Please write me something of great wisdom." The master picks up his brush and paints one word: *Attention*. The student asks "Is that all?" The master writes, *Attention. Attention.*

Attention is concentration elevated above ordinary looking—a focusing of alertness. Without attention we really only live on the surface, yet as automation and machineries have expanded, attention and awareness have receded. The strobe light effect of screen viewing, vibrant flashes of color, light, and sound zap the ability to focus. Children are not born with attention deficit hyperactivity disorders; the environment makes it so. Nurtured on flickering images and noisy devices, the senses cannot sit still. After a lifetime of conditioning, our attention is scattered, and seldom overseen.

The complexity of the mind and nervous system renders our mental processing capacity capable of screening countless bits of information per second. However, our ability to attend consciously is far more limited. Individuals allied with the expansive "right brain" are superior conjurors and multitaskers, more than linear "left brain" thinkers. But when it comes to paying attention, the mind can only truly focus on one thing. Attention is unidirectional, and typically our focus is busy outside in the world, rather than on the light within. Meditation techniques aim to cultivate an inner, one-pointed mind and flow. But the mind is already one-pointed—except its singular focus constantly changes, and our life energies are scattered.

With intention, the mind's lens can be cast wide or narrow. We can direct the mind broadly or closely, out into the world or inside of our own being. When drawn narrow we can appreciate details—thoughts, feelings, gestures, relationships, and foods, and extend loving attention to minute particulars. In this world of distractions and options, a tapered focus can discern the nature of things beyond appearance, belief, or conjecture. Through focused comparison, the rational mind can enter deeply into decisions and arrive at its best understanding. A narrow focus is an excellent way to learn, so long as we remember the whole. When the mind is cast broad it becomes expansive. We can note many things generally and appreciate a fuller perspective. Broad attentiveness and expansive attitudes bless life with deeper meaning. We can appreciate and tune in with aspects of life larger than ourselves.

Awareness

Beyond attention comes *awareness*. Attention is an instrument for survival, manufactured by the mind, and often shifting from idea to idea, perception to perception. In contrast, awareness extends beyond mental processes and is connected to higher consciousness.

Right now, the ideas we have of our "body" are largely (if not wholly) based on data from outside sources. We may scrutinize the data, and the body's exterior, but we seldom really focus within. Modern healthcare systems teach us to know ourselves through symptom diagnosis and expert investigations, carried out in a rational manner. Good scientific research tries to exclude personal views and personal biases. We have been trained to objectify the body, and nullify subjective involvement. Compared with external data, personal experiences and feelings are considered irrational and unworthy. All the while, on the path to embodied eating, feelings of unease

and discomfort are excellent opportunities to learn.

To grow in self-awareness and self-understanding, the living Indian saint Mata Amritanandamayi says that self-awareness does not increase with the acquisition of knowledge, but from the awareness that arises when knowledge accompanies action. Knowledge is *informational* awareness, and embodied eating is *experiential* awareness. To grow we must embody knowledge and live it in our lives. To know ourselves, *Āyurveda* says listen to and observe Mother Nature and Mother Earth; listen to the words of *rishis*, sages, and doctors; listen to the body's wisdom; try knowledge out in your actions; and remain aware.

External, intellectual sources can yield useful information. But a dependence on outside informants forgets the body's natural intelligence and robs us of personal power and personal responsibility. When unaware, life is run by habit and compulsion. To remedy this and grow in inner-awareness, turn the senses toward a more inward-perceiving mode. Direct attention to the body's subtle responses and feelings. Listen and observe. No need to self-reflect or critically analyze. Just witness with fresh eyes, beyond judgements. In touch with awareness there is less compulsion to try to *do* something, working toward outer goals. In fact, awareness is not something you *do*. Awareness is a way of *being*. When we are self-aware, we are both participant and spectator. We are the creator and observer of our own experience. Pausing to apply the light of awareness to habitual thoughts and behaviors can transform mental conflicts and dissolve destructive patterns. Daily acts of food selection, eating, cooking, sitting, moving, communicating, and working are changed.

As inner awareness grows, insights and feelings become touchstones to personal truth and personal choice. We more easily know when something is meaningful or pointless, supportive or best avoided, and make decisions accordingly. Acting in awareness is an antidote to regret. In every situation we do our best within our capacity. A self-aware person is sensitive to the voice of the body, stays in touch with their mental and emotional state, is awake to natural cycles and life around them, and comprehends their place. Through greater self-awareness, our world becomes larger, and our interactions more honest and direct. The more aware we are of what we think, feel, and do, the fuller and purer our life experience. Even if the body is aging or weak, personal awareness can continue to grow.

A Task

Sit in an attitude of relaxed curiosity and simply watch what arises. Rather than look for something, or define what you are looking at, remove all blinkers and lenses, and just watch without expectation or motive. Observe sensations in the food body. Observe if the mind wants to chat or assign meaning. Simply witness thoughts, feelings, emotions.

Our growth as conscious beings is marked not so much by grand gestures, but through the wholehearted awareness we bring. With attention and awareness, the world continues but the way we perceive it alters and deepens.

Observing the Food Body and Mind

At first, the idea of inner observation may seem abstract. We pay a great deal of attention to the food body's external shell, but the interior seems dark and murky. Yet there are many ways to reunite the mind with body and build inner awareness. To observe the food body, first observe each of the five states of matter within you. Observe the actions and qualities of the *dosha*, and their daily cycles. Observe your dominant qualities. Observe the law of cause and effect—the impacts on the body of the world around us and the elements and qualities in the foods you eat. Observe the physical body during activities such as walking, and practices that work across the mind-body system such as yoga, qigong, and tai chi. Observe the breath during physical activity, or during times of stress, hardship, or whenever you think of it. Focusing on the breath is an age-old practice to unite and sensitize the physical and subtle bodies.

Daily we may notice parts of the food body when hunger pangs arise, when eating, when experiencing post-meal satiety, when responding to the call of nature, or if suffering poor physical health. To help regulate why we eat, what foods we eat, and how we eat them, one primary factor is how we know and respond to sensations of hunger and satiation.

Eat According to Hunger—Beware of Imposters

Physical signs of hunger include an empty or rumbling sensation in the belly; a hollow feeling in the gut; mild cramping or distention; difficulty concentrating; lack of energy; a shaky light-headed feeling; irritability; anxiousness; or headache. As well as different symptoms, the experience and intensity of hunger differs among *dosha* types and individuals *Vāta* types tend to have a naturally variable sense of hunger, In imbalanced, *vāta* types become more variable

and capricious, with an appetite that can swing both ways. *Pitta* and mixed *pitta-vāta* individuals tend to experience naturally sharp hunger, and excess *pitta* fires can cause a burning in the gut that is often mistaken as hunger. Those with *kapha* dominance, being heavy and moist by nature, tend to have a slow, low digestion, and experience the least appetite. High *kapha* further smothers the digestive *agni* and suppresses the hunger urge. Across all constitutions, large variations in hunger signals, such as erratic, excessive, or absent hunger points to imbalanced *dosha*, imbalanced digestion, and the likelihood of toxic *āma*. *Āyurveda* understands that excessive and erratic hunger disappears as the *doshas* move toward balance, the toxins are burned and released, and the *agni* settles and strengthens.

Real hunger is not a thought planted by outside sources. When we spend time thinking: *When's lunch? What's for dinner? That looks tasty! Should I have one more piece?* Under these circumstances it's easy to imagine hunger. But rather than begin in the mind, true hunger is a bodily sensation that turns into the thought, *I'm hungry.* According to *Āyurveda*, between four to six hours should pass between meals without undue feelings or thoughts of hunger. For those out of touch, a day of fasting puts us in touch with real hunger. When beginning to observe

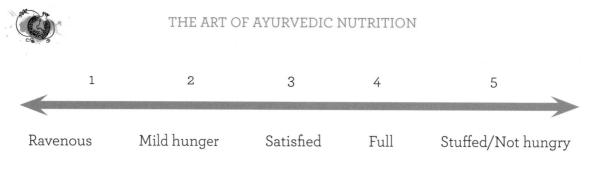

1	2	3	4	5
Ravenous	Mild hunger	Satisfied	Full	Stuffed/Not hungry

Rate your appetite

hunger and satiety it can also be helpful to use a scale. Before, during, and after eating, tune in to how your body really feels, and rate your hunger and satiety. Keeping a record and notes is helpful to identify patterns.

As well as observe hunger, the regulation of hunger and appetite is needed. The best way to synchronize the appetite is to support the food body with regular, nutritious meals that balance the *dosha*. When meals are reliable, hunger pangs are milder, as the body knows it will be fed. When meals are tasty and nourishing, hunger reduces as the cells are comfortably fed. But when the body receives foods dominated by one or two tastes, and those stripped of natural complexity, starved of needed nutrition it is never satisfied. Regulating the appetite (and balancing the *dosha*) is also contingent on balanced digestive fires, so the two must go hand-in-hand. Additional strategies to stabilize hunger include:

- *Manage the environment*. Galvanized to eat, we must become aware of, and learn how to navigate today's plentiful food environment. Rather than viewing commercial food deals and images as potential eating avenues, see them for the sales promotions they are. Don't keep tempting snack foods within easy reach in the home and office.
- *Move the body*. Engaging in physical pursuits stokes digestion, staves off hunger pangs, and invigorates and cleanses the tissues.
- *Breathe deeply*. If we take in more *prāna* through breathing, the food body isn't so reliant or insistent on taking in *prāna* through food.
- *Drink enough water*. Especially in *pitta* types, thirst is commonly mistaken for hunger.
- *Get enough sleep*. Fatigue drives hunger hormones, poor choices, and indigestion.
- *Manage stress*. While acutely stressful events tend to reduce hunger, chronic stress drives hunger. Take steps to minimize, move away from, and effectively

manage ongoing stress. Management strategies include regular walking, sports, yoga, qigong, and mediation; taking a more philosophical perspective; or mustering the courage to make life-changing decisions. When you do experience stress, rather than try to suppress or sedate it, acknowledging the body's stress response helps us manage the situation. Research also suggests that understanding and believing stress is helpful, reduces or even nullifies its negative effects.[18]

Learn to sit with hunger. It's easy to fall prey to eating at the slightest abdominal twinge or an imagined green light. While it's not helpful to become overly hungry, it *is* possible—and beneficial—to sit with mild hunger. Rather than react to hunger in a primal way, explain to the body that food will be forthcoming. Consciously affirm, *I am a little hungry, but I won't eat yet.* Not by force of will, but because it's a conscious choice. This takes self-awareness, and builds mental fortitude and physical endurance. Doing so also helps us better understand our hunger, establish its origin, and ensure we are experiencing a genuine need.

Chew, Chew, Chew

Our teeth give us that winning smile, but their main job is to bite, grind, and break food down.

Conscientious chewing starts the digestive process by breaking down physical and chemical bonds, stimulating the release and mixing of salivary enzymes, facilitating the transformation of food, and telling the *agni* that food is coming. Careful chewing also extends taste and enjoyment and satisfies hunger. The thorough chewing of whole grains, for example, renders them sweeter, lighter, warmer, more digestible, less mucus forming, and more nutritious and satisfying.

If we do not chew each mouthful thirty-two times, we should at least chew each mouthful long enough to liquefy all food. Even heavily processed foods that require little chewing must be mixed with salivary enzymes. So too, medicinal herbs are ideally chewed and mixed with salivary enzymes to optimize absorption. Eating a processed meal only takes five minutes. A home-cooked meal takes ten or fifteen. And enjoying raw foods adds more time again. In order to satisfy hunger and move toward more whole and fresh foods we must relearn the lost art of chewing.

Reduce your usual mouthful, pause with your food, let go of extraneous thoughts, and chew with care and awareness. It takes around twenty minutes for the food body to register fullness. Thorough chewing extends meals, allowing time to register the body's subtle signals. Conscientious chewing means we enjoy food more, and eat less. A pretty good deal for most people.

In order to chew well, the teeth must be in good working order. This is most easily achieved by eating a varied whole food diet that balances the *dosha*; having *kapha* in the birth constitution; no *vāta* or *pitta* imbalance; the support of the genes; good dental hygiene;[12] and visiting a good dentist as (and before) required.

Know Satiation

The term *satiation* refers to feelings of satisfaction or having eaten sufficiently, that bring a meal to its natural end. During a meal as the stomach receives food, physical hunger decreases and internal sensations signal increasing fullness. This transition leads toward a loss in fervor and the slowing and cessation of eating.

While satiation sounds straightforward, many of us are out of touch. The French may consider a meal over when the eater no longer feels hungry, or the food diminishes in flavor or appeal. Americans however, are more influenced by external events. Rather than perceive subtle internal cues, meals are considered done when the beverage runs out, when a "normal" amount has been eaten, or with the cessation of TV watching.[19]

To enhance satiation, become an embodied eater. Observe your meal, eat slowly, chew mindfully, and take note of the body's subtle signals such as growing feelings of heaviness or fullness, a deep breath, reducing interest in food, or a settling burp indicating we have eaten sufficiently. Children taught to finish everything on the plate must work against natural satiety cues.

Eating whole foods high in complexity, roughage, and water offers nutrition and bulk to the stomach that promotes more timely and complete satiation. When we consistently eat smaller meal portions, the stomach—a muscular yet elastic organ—also reduces in size and it takes less food to produce a sense of satiation. For *pitta* types with a sharp hunger, and heavy moist *kapha* individuals, beginning meals with bitter salad greens or raw vegetables such as celery helps to reduce hunger and bring meals to a timely end. Taking around one gram of bitter

---

12   To *Āyurveda*, good dental hygiene includes brushing the teeth first thing in the morning, followed by scraping the tongue, and gargling (swishing, pulling) oil in the mouth for five to fifteen minutes. Known as *gandusha*, regular gargling with sesame (for *vāta* and *kapha*), coconut, or sunflower oil (for *pitta*) is an excellent preventative and remedy for many dental problems.

herbs or the microalgae, spirulina, half an hour before meals can produce a similar effect.

Decode Your Food Cravings

A snack can simply be a snack, but at other times, the urge to eat certain foods or engage in eating behaviors can feel so mammoth that we seemingly have little control. Thoughts and actions fueled by a scrumptious sight or arresting aroma, or unspecified physical, mental, or emotional unrest, take on a life of their own. Sometimes we crave certain tastes, or smooth, crunchy, or liquid textures. Or a specific food, such as chocolate's perfect sweet, fatty, melt-in-the mouth combination. Sometimes the mind craves foods we imagine will bring us pleasure, or at least freedom from pain. From an Ayurvedic perspective, cravings within a robust mind-body system is simply the body asking for constituents it needs. We desire elements, qualities, foods or activities to counter a situation and reinstate balance. Problems arise however, when we don't follow the body's intelligent urges, and when the body becomes impoverished, and imbalance goes too far. Instead of seek what the body requires, we desire substances and actions that actually make us sick. Wayward *vāta* types often crave light, dry foods such as chips and crackers; *pitta* types can crave hot, spicy, oily foods; and *kapha* types yearn for sweet, salty foods such as cakes, cheese,

and biscuits. Hormonal imbalance, which signals *dosha* imbalance, also drives premenstrual yearnings and food cravings.

From a modern nutritional perspective, a lack of minerals such as chromium, magnesium, and zinc can affect insulin metabolism and increase the desire for sweet. Also, being host to errant sugar-loving or acid-loving gut microbes can incite hungers to fulfill their own interests. Those prone to yeast overgrowth and Candida often feel addicted to bread and sugar. And today many foods contain concentrated chemicals that act as drugs. Habitual intakes of coffee, alcohol, refined sugars, fats, salts, food additives, and intense unnatural flavors may offer a rewarding short-term high, but create food addictions and chemical dependencies.[20] In coping with this onslaught, the body does its best to habituate, and soon we need more. Over time, these foods don't make us feel good; but without them we feel worse. Once adapted to junk food, that's what we crave, and natural whole foods don't taste so good.

One antidote to eating habits that don't serve us is to turn eating into a conscious process. Once triggered, the initial seconds of an urge are vital moments when we let compulsion take over, or raise our awareness, and knowingly choose a different path. In the late evening if the mind routinely moves to sweet-seeking mode, rather than reach automatically, look into the thoughts and feelings that have you in their grasp. If a mood gets in the way, switch to observe the mood. A craving for sweet may mean different things, such as: we need to nourish and build up the food body; *dosha* imbalance; hormonal, mineral, or gut flora imbalance; chemical addiction; or perhaps we need sweeter experiences in life. Some food cravings may be satisfied by spending more time in natural beauty, getting a massage, or meeting good friends. Observing an impulse without habitually feeding it begins to eliminate automatic responses and make space for new decisions.

Sometimes we can satisfy a nagging craving by acknowledging, *I'm not hungry, but I'm going to eat anyway.* This declaration places us in a higher state of awareness with more choice of what and how we eat. Then, choose food you truly desire; don't substitute one you think is better for you. Enjoy with all the senses. Remove guilt to defuse the emotional charge. If we know we're making a bad choice, but eat anyway, embodied eaters can observe the effects.

It can be helpful to decode food cravings, but equally, our focus can be best placed on harmonizing the *dosha*, cleansing the system, and eating for health and balance. As eating patterns and lifestyles become more regular, embodied, and balancing, many unhelpful appetites simply fall away. Cleansing and detoxifying the system is another powerful step toward letting go of foods, thoughts, emotions, and behaviors that don't serve us. See Chapter 8 on page 115 for details.

Another Strategy to Know the Food You Eat

Rather than be involved in the eating experience, we have been taught to overthink foods. But with heightened sensitivity and awareness, we can know what a certain food will do for us even before it enters our mouth. By touching, looking at, or lightly contemplating a food, its potential impact can become known. Drawing from the practice of kinesiology, our heart—or rather the vital energy flowing through the heart center—can be a great dietary advisor. We can use this force to test foods and drinks (and also herbs and medicines) we consider taking in.

To begin, stand with your feet together, close your eyes, and become calm and open.

Bend your left arm and hold your upturned palm just below the sternum, where the left and right ribcage meet.

Have an assistant place in your palm the food, fluid, or medicine you wish to test. To "blind" yourself to the food you are holding, have several different foods ready, and keep your eyes closed. To reduce the sensation of touch, the food can be placed on a piece of fabric or card placed on the palm. Packaged substances are okay, but avoid foil and metal.

Stretch the right arm out to the side, tuck the thumb into the palm, and lightly grasp the fingers to make a fist.

Stand quietly and center yourself, then sincerely ask: *is this food good for me right now?*

To test the question, your assistant places their index finger on top of the outstretched right wrist and pushes gently toward the ground.

If the arm can be held stable, the body is energized by the substance, and will benefit.

If, despite a relatively small pressure, the arm moves downward, the system is depleted by the substance, and is best avoided at this time.

Test substances more than once, and retest them over months and years.

Observe the Body's Wastes

Most of us pay little attention to the wastes we excrete. We have a basic idea of "normal", and spray air fresheners and open windows. Although not a subject for most dinner table conversations, waste production and removal are vital functions. All physical metabolism creates unneeded by-products that must be removed. If not, they build up, pollute the system, weaken the immunity, and usher in disease. In contrast, effective waste removal keeps the food body clean and every aspect of health supported. According to *Āyurveda*, the body's wastes include feces; urine; sweat; excreta of the ears, eyes, nose, mouth, and genitals; body hair; and nails, all of which are well worth contemplating. Through normal metabolic processes, additional *doshas* are produced inside the body and must also be eliminated. Excess *vāta* is expelled as gas and through muscular and nervous energy; excess *pitta* through bile and acids; excess *kapha* as mucus. After excess *dosha*, the three main wastes *Āyurveda* considers are feces, urine, and sweat.

Overall, our natal constitution directs what we as individuals should consider *normal*. Knowledge about quantity, qualities, frequency, and ease can indicate natal constitution, or signpost *dosha* imbalance. Daily inspection shows us the effects of various food and lifestyle choices, tells us how the metabolism is functioning, and supports health-oriented decisions. To attend to our wastes, we can hone all of the senses, but in general, sight, smell, and hearing suffice.

Observe the Feces

Feces are the body's way of disposing solid waste. From a Western perspective, the bulk of stool consists of plant roughage and the bodies of trillions of bacteria. From an Ayurvedic view, stool is mainly excess earth and water. As well as waste removal, feces provides temporary strength and tone to the lower abdomen and colon. The colon is the home base of *vāta dosha* and anchors it in place. All problems concerning the feces involve and disrupt *vāta dosha*. Before we look at indications of imbalance, let's consider general signs of healthy stool.

Indications of a Healthy Stool

- Voiding the bowels first thing in the morning a short time after waking
- Light to medium brown, to tan or yellowish in color
- Complete evacuation with no residual sensation or discomfort
- The shape and density of a ripe banana
- A smooth diameter without bumps, indentations, and twisting
- Minimal presence of undigested food
- Not overly smelly
- Floats just below the water's surface

From these general indications, our birth constitution influences what is normal, plus the influence of any current *dosha* imbalance. In general, those with *vāta* dominance tend toward smaller volumes. The stool is harder, drier, and can be darker in color. Small pebble-sized feces can form, and dry constipation is a tendency. Evacuation likely occurs once a day, and copious gas can be passed without much odor. Excess *vāta* creates irregular, rough, or pellet-shaped stool, and symptoms such as intermittent spasm, bubbling gas, bloating, painful, or incomplete elimination, constipation, and fluctuations from constipation to diarrhea—otherwise known as irritable bowel syndrome (IBS). A stool that floats like a boat implies too much air element is present.

In health, *pitta*-dominant individuals generally void larger, softer volumes that can be smelly and tend toward yellowish, and the bowels open two or three times daily. In *pitta* excess, the feces can become very yellow or green in color, and the elimination can be especially splashy, accompanied by burning or surplus odor. An inflamed bowel is also a sign of *pitta* aggravation. Symptoms can include diarrhea (especially if stressed, or after hot, spicy foods), an urgency to get to the bathroom (but sometimes passing very little), blood or pus in the stool, feelings of burning and incomplete evacuation, and abdominal distention and pain.

In *kapha* domination, heavy, dense stools are usually passed once a day—a ritual that can require some sitting. The excreta can be lighter in color, and may smell slightly milky or sweet. Mucus can be present. In *kapha* excess, the stool becomes heavier, and constipation and feelings of stuckness occur; a morning coffee, hot meal, cigarette, or laxative is needed to kick-start the motor. For all *dosha* types, strong smelling, sinking, sticky feces are a sign that *āma* is present. Check how much toilet paper you use.

Other influences on stool volume, color, and consistency include the foods we eat. In general, fruits and vegetables are designed to cleanse and leave the body. Eating more fruits and vegetables increases the volume of the stool. And naturally pigmented foods such as carrots, spinach, and beets contribute their colors to the mix. Whole grains are designed to nourish and stay in the body. Eating more grains and especially refined ones, support smaller, fewer bowel movements. Meat, being heavy, dense, and devoid of dietary fiber also contributes to solid, infrequent stools. Very dark or black stools signify the presence of iron from the diet or blood in the gastrointestinal tract, or the presence of *āma*. During extended cleansing, as toxins leave deeper tissues and reenter the gut, stool can become smellier and stickier, a positive sign of detoxification.

At this time the tongue, too, can become more coated and furrier.

To support regular bowels, do the following:

- Consume whole foods (especially fruits and vegetables) that support your constitution
- Eat meals balanced in taste, and choose food combinations that are readily digested
- Nurture healthy gut microbes
- Drink adequate fluids, and eat adequate natural oils and oily foods. Warm water and most oils are natural laxatives
- Nurture a regular eating pattern and daily routine that involves physical activity
- Avoid too much worry, fear, and other withering, contracting emotions including frigidity and attachment
- Don't use and abuse laxatives, colonic irrigation, coffee, drugs, or antibiotics
- If still constipated try one or both of the following: take two to four teaspoons of psyllium husk in the morning with plenty of warm water; take one to two teaspoons of *triphala* powder with warm water at night, just before bed.

With time and persistence, a pattern of bowel regularity forms.

Stick Out Your Tongue

The tongue's surface provides an excellent indication of the state of the *dosha* inside the gut, and which *dosha* is causing a problem. First thing in the morning a thin film of dead bacteria on the tongue is normal, but a thick, textured, or colored coating indicates *dosha* imbalance and *āma* in the digestive system. When the tongue is protruded, the back third corresponds to the colon and *vāta dosha*, the middle third to the small intestine and *pitta dosha*, and the third nearest the tip to the stomach and *kapha dosha*. A thick coating at the back, middle, or tip of the tongue indicates *āma* in the colon, small intestine, or stomach/thorax, respectively. A coating over two thirds or all of the tongue indicates multiple *dosha* are involved. During detoxification, the covering on the tongue can become very thick as toxins reenter the digestive system for release.

The color of the coating also offers clues. *Āma* mixed with *vāta* presents as a thin, dry coating that can range from pale to dull, or sometimes blackish-brown or purplish in color. *Āma* mixed with *pitta* is a moderate yellow or greenish coating. Red tongue patches, excessive shininess, and inflammation are additional signs of high *pitta*. On the tongue, *āma* mixed with *kapha dosha* tends to be thick, white, and matte or shiny. Other diagnostic clues include a rough or cracked tongue indicating internal dryness from excess *vāta*, and ridges or tooth imprints lining the front edges of the tongue indicating nutrient malabsorption in the gut.

Observe Your Waterworks

Producing and passing urine is the food body's primary way to remove excess water element, maintain fluid homeostasis, and excrete surplus heat of the fire element including acid wastes. Every day, the amount of urine we produce depends on *dosha* type and balance, plus how much fluid we drink, eat, sweat, and eliminate as feces. In *vāta* individuals, urine is usually light in color or clear, and more frequent but less in quantity. In *vāta*-aggravation, the need to urinate small volumes can disrupt sleep and other activities. *Pitta* types require more fluids, and often pass high quantities of urine. Pure *pitta* types and those with excess *pitta* can pass urine with a strong yellow color and pungent odor. *Kapha* dominance can create opaque or cloudy urine that is more alkaline, and may be sweet-smelling, or harbor mucus. Our waterworks are also affected by fluids, foods, herbs, and other medicines and actions either for the better or the worse. In particular, drinking too little, drinking too much—especially cold and aerated drinks, and alcohol—the use of diuretic drugs, excess sex, stress, and emotional shock upset the water-works and *imbalance vāta* and *kapha doshas*.

Sweat It Out

Similar to feces and urine, sweat serves more than one purpose. According to *Āyurveda*, sweating removes excess fire and water, is a waste product of the metabolism of fat, an alternative channel to the bladder and bowel to remove the soluble wastes, a way to manage body temperature and cool the system, a vehicle to nourish and lubricate the skin, and a way to reduce heaviness and stiffness in the body. While feces and urine must be released regularly, sweating only occurs when body temperature rises. Those with *pitta* dominance tend to sweat the most—a perspiration that can stain yellow and smell malodorous. *Kapha* types can sweat a moderate amount—more if there is *kapha* excess. *Vāta* types may sweat very little and suffer from dry, cracked skin, especially when unbalanced.

The body's sweat mechanisms can be damaged through excessive use of saunas, Jacuzzis, hammams, and sweat lodges; overuse of drugs or herbs that induce sweating; too many dry foods; lack of good quality salts; and too much or too little exercise. According to *Āyurveda*, the processes of sweating and digestion are linked. When the body produces sweat, the digestive

fires rest. (One reason why exercise suppresses appetite.)

Awaken and Manage the Senses

All plants and animals have sense organs, and through their unique sensory capacities every being perceives its own worldview. For humans, the five sense organs—the eyes, ears, nose, tongue, and skin—are our primary windows to personally see, hear, smell, taste, and touch or feel our outer and inner world. Conceptually the sense impulses come into the head because four of five sense organs are located there—but the senses permeate the body. What we take into the body as sense impressions affects and conditions the psychology, and by association, the physical body. Today, the sense of sight dominates our perceptions. Through sight we evaluate; construct charts and diagrams to see what's possible; imagine in our mind's eye. When it comes to eating, the sight of food powerfully stimulates or repulses before taste, smell, touch, or hunger enter the equation. But sight, as well as our other sense perceptions, can be deceived.

Our windows of perception are delicate structures, yet much about modern life tortures and dulls the senses, and pays no mind to sense control. At best, we are taught to organize the sensory impressions we take in from outside—to label and assign relative worth. Plus, just as the food we eat conditions the metabolism, the sense impressions we take in condition the mind. Rather than nurture sensory scope and acuity, the senses are confined to a narrow, biased, outward-bound range—while the core of sensory experience lies within us. To awaken, sharpen, and govern the senses and enhance our ability to receive life as it is, one primary practice is to begin to consciously choose what we pay attention to, and what we ignore. Rather than indiscriminate windows, the mind's senses should act as sentinels in a selection and rejection role, choosing which impressions to bring in, and which to reject. Protecting ourselves from undesirable impressions reduces the *rajas* and *tamas* we bring in, promotes *sattva* and natural intelligence, and rests and rejuvenates the mind. Rather than limiting or dulling down the senses, yoga traditions talk about controlling, withdrawing, and detaching the senses from the external world, and directing our focus within.

To nurture and invigorate the senses, spend time in Mother Nature, and sincerely appreciate and contemplate beautiful things. Imbibe wonderful aromas; absorb full and balanced flavors; hear great words and music; keep the skin supple and soft. When the senses no longer run amok, we are naturally more receptive and responsive to life's elements, qualities, and cycles. Making the right choice in the right moment becomes straightforward.

Observe and Manage the Mind

We tend to think of the brain as the mind, but *Āyurveda* and yoga understand that the field through which our thoughts move permeates throughout and expands beyond physical body to wherever we consciously focus. The physical body is the vessel of the mind—the material structure through which the mind perceives, experiences, and acts. In this way, the physical body is a gross aspect of the mind, and the mind is a subtle aspect of the body. Vedic scriptures liken the mind-body relationship to milk in a copper pot. The milk (the mind) readily takes on the shape and characteristics of the vessel (the body). Rather than distinct entities, the body and mind are functionally integral.

As the food body provides the structure, our physical constitution greatly influences mental functions. Light, airy *vāta dosha* motivates mental movement and desire for stimulation and change. *Vāta* and *vāta* dual types tend to be more curious, creative, and likely to try new things. Out of balance they can be capricious and forgetful. *Pitta's* primary qualities of warmth, light, intensity, and ability to spread, lend themselves to courageous, goal-oriented psychologies that love achievement and challenge. Out of balance they can be angry and intimidating, just as too many spicy foods breed hot, fiery emotions. *Kapha dosha*, dominated by heavy, stable, slow attributes nurtures a robust, caring mental constitution that seeks permanence and security, but in imbalance can become bogged down, dull, and depressive, just as heavy foods breed heavy thoughts.

However, over and above our physical constitution, it is the three great cosmic qualities—*sattva, rajas,* and *tamas*—that overlie all mental functions and primarily influence the mind. *Sattva* creates intelligence, clarity, understanding, honesty, openness, flexibility, caring, and joy, and is a stabilizing force. *Rajas* drives expansion and curiosity, keeps thoughts and emotions flowing, and in excess creates agitation, frustration, impatience, hyperactivity, anger, and aggression. *Tamas* brings heaviness, coolness, and restriction, and holds mental processes in check. Excessive *tamas* creates mental rigidity and dullness, concealment, repression, manipulation, delusion, and depression.

The mind is sensitive enough to perceive and project countless substantial and subtle phenomena. But as a sensitive energy field, the mind is a delicate organ. The mental sheath is sensitive to incoming foods, through their effects on food body and *dosha*, and through the *sattva, rajas,* and *tamas* we take in. In addition to tastes and combinations that imbalance the *dosha*, general food habits that imbalance and desensitize the mind include consuming too much coffee and alcohol; too many spicy and rich foods; too many refined sugars and oils; meals that are too large, too late, too many mixed ingredients, or contain foods that are foreign to the food body.

The mind also influences the physical body—every thought and emotion elicit biological change. Patterns of thought create patterns in the metabolism and physiology. If the mind is calm, the body is calm. If thoughts are racing, how can the body sit still? Repetitive thoughts harboring fears, worries, jealousies, hates, and angers damage the mind's delicate balance, trigger mistakes of the intellect, or *prājñāparādha*, and cause physical unease. When the mind is not balanced it upsets, and is upset by, emotional, sensorial, and physical phenomena. But even though our thoughts and emotions are influenced by untold inner and outer events, we must take responsibility for them.

To characterize and *know* the mind, Vedic, Yogic, and Buddhist traditions view thoughts as the mind's objects. The mind is subtle, yet we can observe its contents—thoughts, impressions, emotions—as objects passing through the mental field. To view the mind's contents as objects passing through helps the ego-mind detach, the aspect of mind that owns and perpetuates our personality. Seeing thoughts and emotions as objects creates distance from mental constructs so we can begin to disentangle ourselves, and see more plainly and clearly. To begin to observe the mind's objects try one or more of the following suggestions.

- Whenever it occurs to you, watch where the mind goes. What subjects and thoughts dominate? How many ideas are positive and reinforcing? How many are unconstructive or dull?
- Notice when the mind makes comparisons and judgements.
- Take time to notice your sense organs, and observe what they take in.
- Listen to your self-talk. Is it self-deprecating? Self-serving? Supportive? Hear also what you say to others.
- Look at what motivates recurrent fears, insecurities, and desires.
- Notice passing moods and emotions. To be attentive you don't need to be peaceful. With practice, we can be aware

in the midst of a raging fury, conscious of the dissonance of uncomfortable decisions. Observe arising emotions as objects.
- Notice signs of *rajas* and *tamas*.
- Observe the imagination at play, glorifying past memories and future dreams.
- Observe the mind's influence on the body's responses and actions. How the mind thinks, the physiology responds the same way.
- Even if the mind is muddled, just begin to observe. Knowing that the mind is muddled is a type of clarity!

Neither the mind nor body evolved to live in today's urban societies. Yet, our success and well-being in this world in large part depends on our ability to unite and harness the prowess of the mind-body system. The physical body is the structure through which the mind expresses itself, and the mind's subtle energies influence the physical body's formation and plight. If the mind alone seeks benefits and pleasure, the body goes to hospital. Only when the mind acts in service of the body can we fully process knowledge and create understanding through personal experience.

Living Experience

Many words are offered to help us describe what's happening in the body, fathom life, and make choices, but nothing clarifies understanding like firsthand, personal experience. Gautama Buddha told his followers, here are the teachings, go and try them for yourself. Along the Buddhist path, developing wisdom and knowing through experience is one of six steps to spiritual union. In Hinduism, the *Atharva Veda* says do not be led by others, awaken your own mind, amass your own experience, and decide for yourself your own path. The link between knowledge and experience is continuous and dynamic. Only by experiencing our own path can we be happy and make our fullest contribution.

Day and night, modern life invites us to buy, try, and experience new things. Yet this involvement is largely outbound and shallow. Rather than be satisfied with superficialities, to reclaim life's experiences we must learn to sense and feel deeply. True experience lies within. When it comes to food and eating choices, involve your whole self in looking, listening, tasting, smelling, and feeling your way. Prepare your eating area. Notice the qualities in the places and spaces where you prepare food and eat. Do your best to remove distractions such as televisions, loud music, and computers. Prioritize fresh air and natural light. Sit still, and if possible, face east in the direction of the rising sun, our source of fire, heat, and light. Chew each mouthful carefully and experience the fullness of flavors and textures—crunchy, chunky, gritty, stringy, creamy. Close the eyes to focus attention and awareness.

A Task

Contemplate a single food, such as a peanut or sultana. Sit down and hold it in your palm. Observe it deeply, take time to ponder its source, consider its willingness to be incorporated into your own body, be with emotions and feelings that arise. Then, slowly eat it, appreciating its numerous qualities, and humbly giving thanks.

Sometimes eat a plated meal using your hands. Transferring food to mouth via the fingertips activates physical and subtle pathways, offers temperature and textural cues and, many Indians agree, enhances taste. After meals, remain receptive to qualities manifesting in the body, such as heating or cooling, or moistening or drying effects.

Choosing where we focus, turning the senses inward, and consciously experiencing cultivate deeper awareness and sensitivity to better understand ourselves and our place in the world, and the foods we eat and their influence on our system.

Feel Your Way

All life *feels*. Early last century, the famous Indian biologist, physicist, and botanist, Sir Jagadish Chandra Bose, confirmed that plants possess sense organs, and can perceive touch, light, heat, cold, sound vibrations, and other external stimuli.[21] Plants can also perceive predators and potential threats, not only when physically present, but communicated through thought or intention.[22] For *Āyurveda*, plants have internal consciousness, and a soul. Animals also feel, and so do their seemingly simple products, such as yogurt and eggs. Experiments using a polygraph machine documented a fear reaction in eleven eggs after the first of the dozen was cracked; and a distress response in yogurt when injected with penicillin to kill bacteria.[23] One more reason to handle the foods we eat gently, and with gratitude and respect.

Among human beings, Carl Jung described *feeling* as an essential condensation of energy that can be perceived internally, and talked about a feeling-tone.[24] Feelings are the movement of *prāna*; vibrations, sometimes pleasant, sometimes not, that can be perceived. Without feeling, life is dry and mechanical. With feeling, life has more juice. Developing inner sensitivity to deep feelings provides new ways of knowing ourselves and the world we live in. Through conscious feeling we feel things in ourselves and feel ourselves in things. We can feel empathy and compassion for others, who just like us have frailties and limitations. More than our physical actions, it's the feelings we experience that impress themselves upon us. By following feelings when making small and big decisions we change our path. It's empowering to know how you feel!

To awaken feeling, develop the mind's powers of observation, and pay attention to the body, especially the sense of touch. Touch is present from the beginning of life, pervades the whole body, and is seen by *Āyurveda* as foundational for the other four senses. Touch perceives the elements of air, fire, water, and earth; and qualities including hot, cold; smooth, rough; heavy, light; hard, soft; solid, liquid; pleasant, painful; hunger, thirst; and impulsion and mobility. Feel the elements and qualities that are dominant in you. Notice gut reactions. Pay attention to the heart, and turn to face your deepest feelings. But don't think too much. The way you think is the way you feel. If the mind is sad, the body is sad too. If the mind is courageous and enthusiastic, the body lines up these feelings too. Nothing disturbs feelings so much as thoughts. Put aside rational thinking and analysis, and simply feel your way. After the brain the gut is the most enervated area of the body. When relaxed and comfortable the gut's reaction to foods, meals, ideas, and circumstances are excellent clues, especially when things don't feel right.

As well as the movement of time, the mind and its senses, and the *doshas* and gut, the heart is another fundamental point where disease can commence or be healed. Nowhere in the body feels more fiercely than the heart. *Āyurveda* considers the mind and senses have their roots in the heart. When our heart is open and we are relaxed, heartfelt feelings reveal our truest insights and nature. Acting on heartfelt feelings and desires generates happiness and meaning in life. Deep feelings of love, forgiveness, and compassion toward others and ourselves, support and hasten healing. Rather than assert your will and work through the ego, let the force of the heart rise up. To awaken feeling, lie beneath the stars and let the moon's cool light in. Absorb the radiance of the sun's morning rays. Walk barefoot on the grass; sit beside a flower and bear witness; breathe in the fragrance and freshness of spring. Delight in food. Enjoyment, gratitude, and contentment are great digestive aids. Move with feeling. Practice yoga postures, breath expansion and control (*prānāyāma*), tai chi and qigong to energize and unify the mind and body, and awaken graceful expression and flow. Allow life to flow through every part. No words, no thoughts—only feelings. Feel beauty. Slow down. Relax more. Meditate when you can.

It's possible to collect information upon information, knowledge upon knowledge, and yet never digest and understand. What we gather is our own, and it's up to us what we do with it. We can collect experience upon experience, and feeling upon feeling, and still fail to learn. Don't mix up feelings and emotions. Emotions are of the mind, and often socially implanted. Feelings are more visceral. Our deepest feelings are less affected by society, generally last longer, and are ultimately more real. When feelings spark inner knowing, it is our challenge to notice and respond. As the body is given a voice, the mind must be willing to honor its feelings and support the body's intelligence. Who knows how you feel, except you? Let personal experience and feeling become your guiding light.

Develop Your Sixth Sense

Vedic scriptures speak of the five senses, and also a sixth sense or inner voice. This inner expression is not the conscience, and does not depend on the mind or senses. It is an inner intelligence or knowing originating outside of conscious processes, received in the physical body or through higher awareness. The inner voice emerges as a sudden gut hunch, as deep feelings of discomfort, as an upwelling in the heart, or moment of clear insight or understanding. Jung explained intuition as the inner occurrence of something odd, outside the mind's comprehension. Osho called this inner expression the wordless voice of understanding deep within the heart; an inner knowing tuned to the universe that speaks when all other voices are silent. Intuition does not need a preceding thought, and is an excellent opportunity to learn, free from past ideas and biases. When there is knowing, but no concept of how or why, the inner voice has spoken.

Cultivating your inner guidance system is an imperative accessory for life, and also for eating. Being perceptive and responsive to inner knowing allows decisions to be made free from mental mistakes and misconceptions. When the mind allows it, intuition can guide the body and deeper-self toward a certain choice or path. Other times we are warned against paths we best not take—what not to eat, what not to do, where not to go. If heeded, these warnings avoid much trouble. Intuitive guidance can also be passive in nature. The Indian sage Sri Aurobindo called the intuitive mind a way of being, where we wait to perceive our inner voice before acting on anything of consequence. Be quiet and do nothing until, when the time is right, the inner voice guides decisions and actions.

The inner voice is most audible when we live in stable circumstances and environments, according to Nature's cycles; eat a natural, *dosha*-friendly diet; cleanse and rejuvenate as required; nurture attention, awareness, and feeling; and are quiet, relaxed, open, and sincere. Sometimes intuition is fostered through repeating skills or experiences. Insights can also be accessed through complete attention and presence, fully tuning into situations. Other times inner knowing rises through the sagacity of collective wisdom. Insights also happen when we hit rock bottom, bubbling up through sheer force, or when we finally let go. In illness, deep inner guidance is often present, but we are too overwhelmed to be alerted to problems or courses of action. Or we are too busy overanalyzing and asking for *proof* before we respond. During upheaval and emotional crisis dreams of an intuitive nature often occur.

Conscious Cookery

As a society, we have been conditioned to believe that home-cooked meals are effort and time wasted. But time taken to prepare and cook food is an investment in our health and the health of those we cook for. We don't lose time by home cooking, or sitting down to enjoy a meal. Endeavors to plan and eat wholesome foods reward us and our loved ones with vitality now, and future health and well-being. Plus, the processes of food acquisition, preparation, cooking, and eating provide important opportunities to interact with and augment the life and qualities of the foods we consume. Be a conscious shopper, cook, and consumer. And involve children to nurture appreciation of fresh whole foods, and miracles of taste and transformation.

Cooking is commonly the first stage of digestion. Processes such as soaking, chopping, grating, grinding, and heating soften food, break down physical and chemical bonds, and create smaller components that are easier to eat and digest. While some vitality and nutrients are lost during cooking, improved digestibility generally outweighs this loss.

Through cooking we come in contact with the elements of earth, water, fire, and air, and different cooking methods benefit different *dosha*. Baking and dry-roasting dry up water and contract tissues (earth). In order to digest these foods, the body must add moisture back. Drying cooking methods can help pacify *kapha* dominance, but adversely affect *vāta dosha*. Moist cooking methods, such as steaming, stewing, and soups maintain and augment the water element, which support internal moisture and *vāta dosha*. Foods cooked together in a liquid medium such

as a one-pot stew, blend and soften in qualities and actions, and are easier to assimilate than the same foods cooked separately. Soups and stews are useful for those with weak digestion, internal dryness, fragile teeth, chronic illness, and during rejuvenation therapy. All cooking adds the element of fire to food (especially if cooked over a flame), and supports the digestive fires. This warmth is especially beneficial for *vāta* types, but consuming foods and drinks that are too hot can destroy *vāta's* strength. As cooking introduces heat, *pitta*-dominant individuals should allow cooked foods to cool a little before eating, and can benefit by including raw foods.

Of course, the ingredients we choose also contribute their qualities. Herbs and spices are concentrated foods that add their tastes, aromas, attributes, actions, colors, and textures to meals. Through their use we can enliven and balance meals, and also use them to antidote unwanted qualities. *Kapha* types, for example, can introduce the warm, dry qualities of chili to a moist, heavy dish. Or *vāta* types can grate some ginger over a meal to bring heat, freshness, and give digestion a boost. *Pitta* types can add generous quantities of bitter, astringent herbs such as cilantro and parsley over warmer, spicier meals. Recipes can also be modified to reduce or exclude aggravating foods, or include pacifying foods.

Further considerations include:

- Cooking over a gas flame is preferable to electric hot plates.
- Don't overcook foods, or use long, forceful cooking methods unnecessarily. Prefer fast methods such as steaming and stir frying, or slow, gentle simmering.
- When cooking, foster patience. Be expedient with your techniques, but take time to create full, balanced flavors.
- Cooked food is considered *fresh* for one-and-a-half hours.
- Eating well-stored and re-prepared leftovers is preferable to fast foods or a microwave meal. Store leftovers in the fridge in a glass or non-reactive container, and consume within one day. Once cooled in the fridge or freezer, meals become drier and harder to digest, and more prone to aggravate *vāta*. Add extra digestive spices, moisture, and/or *ghee*. Reheat gently and fully.
- Plastic vessels for storage, eating, and drinking transfer plastic residues into food and should be avoided. *Āyurveda* prefers ceramic, glass, or stainless steel. Traditionally, gold vessels are recommended for *vāta*, silver for *pitta*, and bronze or copper for *kapha*.

- Avoid microwave ovens. The application of microwaves may seem convenient, but irreparably damages food, rendering it foreign to the body. Never heat baby's milk or food in a microwave oven.
- Avoid eating at places where meals are mass-produced and reheated.

Conscious cookery is an ideal opportunity to nurture our relationship with food. At all times, handle food with good intentions, and nurture respect for the food and the needs of those who will eat it. Through conscious participation we render the whole greater than the sum of its parts.

Our Food Relations

Ancient Vedic texts understand food as the first born among all beings. All that exists on earth is born of food, lives on food, and in the end merges into food. Food is the universal medicine.[25] To enable and sustain life on Earth, food is an offering from the gods. Consciously acknowledging this gift, and food's central role, is an imperative part of sentient, embodied eating. So that we may live, the act of eating requires that other animals and plants must die. Truly appreciating the cyclical nature of eating nurtures awareness and compassion, helps to harmonize the foods we eat, and reduces potential negative effects on us, and the wider environment. Whether elaborate or modest, store-bought or homemade, be respectful of and thankful for the foods and water you have access to, and the meals produced.

How we recognize and appreciate the foods we eat is entirely personal. Say and do whatever feels meaningful and conveys your sentiment. Some thank God or Mother Nature, or their form of divine creator. We can thank Mother Earth for her bounty; acknowledge the vital contributions of the five great elements, and sun and moon. We also owe a debt of gratitude to countless soil microbes, pollinating insects, and human beings. Meals or medicines prepared and received amid prayers are powerful healing entities. Still heard in India, this Sanskrit invocation sung at communal gatherings honors food and its effects, and asks that all beings be fulfilled and happy. It translates to:

Let us be together. Let us eat together.
Let us produce energy together.
Let there be no limit to our energies.
Let there be no ill feeling among us.
Om ... Peace, Peace, Peace.

To deepen our food relations and become a flexible, responsive eater we simply need to pay more attention, remain aware, and live each eating experience. Following guidance also requires a willingness to act on insights without constantly overanalyzing or seeking validation. Embodied eating involves the physical body and its five elements, the mind and its senses, the movement of *prāna* and feeling, intuitive wisdom, and the heart and soul. The more you listen, respond, and experience, the more you learn.

CHAPTER 11

Satmya: Habituation and Habits

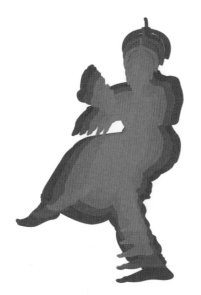

Pay attention to every body, every day!

Living biological systems are arranged in repeating patterns. Repetition is an intrinsic foundation of cosmic and human nature. In the past, food habits were largely dictated by seasonal cycles and recurring religious and social rituals. Today, life continues to revolve around repetition of celestial and communal events, albeit with less meaningful ceremony and seasonal rhythm. Over our lifetime, repetitive food habits develop through upbringing, schooling, peer groups, food advertising and media, and through personal experiences, preferences, and tendencies. And these acquired food routines, lingos, symbols, and beliefs insert meaning into the meals we eat.

Throughout life we create habits, then become habituated to them. This habituation can take a positive or negative turn. In the positive, habituation or *satmya* is one way the food body moves toward balance. With time and repetition, the body can adjust to contact with different foods, climates, and situations, yet this can take years or generations. Those who emigrate to a new country may never feel adapted. Living within local seasons and eating locally grown produce enhances acclimatization. The food body can even adapt to an over-processed denatured diet. If habituated to unwholesome foods or drugs (or if taken in small quantity, or the digestive power or constitution is strong), less harm occurs. But habituation to noxious foods or drugs may also result in alteration of the natural metabolism. Toxins are tucked away in deep tissues, so life can continue immediately, but long-term disease is created. Being habituated to unwholesome foods or only one or two tastes is an inferior type of *satmya*. Superior *satmya* is to be accustomed to fresh, local meals containing all six tastes.

Entertaining the same ideas and behaviors activates and strengthens metabolic pathways. By engaging in a regular rhythm of eating, the body prepares to receive familiar food. Similar for sleep; a reliable, *dosha*-friendly bedtime lays a foundation for rejuvenating slumber. By adapting to repeated thoughts and actions, less stress is placed on the system; practices become easier,

more efficient, and reinforced. The process of adaptation and habituation keeps the body alive, and if the circumstances allow, to thrive. Habituation is intelligence at work. Selected, organized practices also serve as reference points from which we can operate that protect the *doshas* when exposed to sudden shocks or stressors.

In the negative, practices that become easier and more efficient often become mindless too. Becoming habituated to habits enables thoughts and activities to take place without conscious decision. When our eating scripts run somewhere low in awareness, food choice becomes an automatic behavior that ignores personal responsibility. External forces dictate, and we lose the freedom to respond to different situations. When it comes to food, we are born with *neo-phobia*, a built-in negativity bias that makes us more likely to see new foods as "bad," rather than "good." We enjoy familiarity, fear unknown tastes, and have an inborn preference for sweets, salts, and fats—alongside a commercial food supply that acts as addictive drugs. *Āyurveda* understands the trapping of actions in time as a prime cause of suffering that become barriers to be crossed. Old routines perpetuate painful cycles, discount creativity and future options, and obstruct change and balance. The extent to which we can live with bad habits depends on our daily dosage, and how detrimental they are to our birth constitution.

Daily habits can break us or make us. When our core ideas and behaviors are advantageous, our entire being prospers. Supportive routines and habits that complement our surroundings and constitution act as life's best affirmations. And yet, whatever we do and keep on doing, increases our affinity to do the same thing again. In this way, unsupportive habits carry us far from a balanced state. Becoming conscious of unfavorable habits provides an opportunity to move closer to balance. Then, new choices must be exercised, and new pathways forged. This chapter considers the process of habit change, including physical and mental practices to support the release of old unfavorable habits, and establish habits that are new and advantageous.

Preparing for Habit Change

During infancy and childhood, the body is like wet clay. The impressions we take in create new pathways, but by adulthood the clay is dry. Then, instead of efficient creation, the system focuses on maintaining developed routes and letting unused pathways fall away. This is another reason why old and often repeated habits are difficult to erase, and it's not easy to forge new paths.

Long-standing habits naturally feel hardwired, yet this is not the case. Each decision made for change shifts nerve impulses in another direction.

In Western sociology and behavioral psychology, one model used to explain behavior change is the social cognitive theory, which understands that people and their environment grow together, and behaviors result from this interaction.[26] To motivate change, environments must be in some way supportive, and accompanied by personal factors including our capacity to foresee positive outcomes of a new behavior; whether we possess the necessary knowledge, skills, and confidence to perform it; and whether we possess problem-solving skills to cope with emotions and barriers that arise.

Our birth constitution and present *dosha* imbalance can also affect our ability to change. *Vāta* dominance can create attitudes that are unfixed and impulsive. Especially when unbalanced, this can undermine long-lasting change and the adoption of beneficial habits. A balanced *pitta* constitution can illuminate harmful habits and take committed steps to transform. Yet the sharp, spreading nature of *pitta dosha* can also perpetuate debilitating habits, or attempt overly radical change. *Kapha* types like routine, can struggle to let go of old habits, and least enjoy change. But once in motion, they can treat obstacles as stepping-stones rather than barriers, and build and maintain new habits well.

For all constitutions, if *rajas* governs the psychology, focus can be difficult, and tangible results are often required or the mind simply moves on. When *tamas* rules, change and adaptation stagnate. In a *tamasic* mind for progress to be made, the stimulation of *rajas* is needed, plus additional motivation and support. In *sattva* dominance, intelligent choices are easy and adaptation and harmonious change can occur. Rather than rush in, *sattvic* individuals choose their time, and work in concert with the environment.

It's easy to fill ourselves and our lives with thoughts, foods, qualities, and actions, but difficult to empty them out. Transition starts with greater awareness of the habits that don't serve us. Our task is then to let go of old unbalanced habits to make room for the new.

Just Let Go
Change may seem random, but it's actually an inherently ordered process. Across space and time, something retreats and something expands; something dissolves and something grows; regeneration comes from decay. The medicine

of negation is a powerful tool in dietary change, and in life. In order to introduce new foods and behaviors, first recognize, reduce, and eliminate what's of no use. Shedding what is no longer needed generates clarity and room to grow. Life at its core is a continual letting go. In order to let go of unfavorable dietary and lifestyle habits, consider these additional things worth dropping:

- To help shed what's past and remain open to the future, let go of *knowing*. We may see life in terms of black and white, but sometimes what's right turns out to be wrong, and bad decisions often work out for the best. Don't hold rigid unquestioned beliefs or cling to what you think you know. Inquiry stops when we believe. Sadhguru, the living Indian yogi and mystic says, rather than identify with your knowledge, which is inherently limited; identify with your ignorance, which is boundless. Welcome the unknown. Make space for exploration and learning.
- Let go of *fear*. Fear is normal and sometimes helpful, but observe how fear affects the mind, and how we act under its influence. Look your fears in the face, and let irrational ideas go. Leave your comfort zone, lest it becomes your prison.

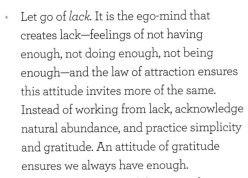

- Let go of *lack*. It is the ego-mind that creates lack—feelings of not having enough, not doing enough, not being enough—and the law of attraction ensures this attitude invites more of the same. Instead of working from lack, acknowledge natural abundance, and practice simplicity and gratitude. An attitude of gratitude ensures we always have enough.

- Let go of *desiring*. In life, most often we are given what we need—maybe not all we desire—but what we need to live and grow. Desires often form the seeds of disease. When the mind drops its attachments and accepts its present state, the emotions and physical body are set free.

- Let go of *the need to feel in control*. The thoughts and structures that guide and define us also limit our freedom. Life is not precise; it has nuance and self-expression. By understanding our complete interdependence with the world, the question of control ceases. The more we let go of the need to control and simply observe what is, the more power we have.

- Let go of *being the doer*. In the *Bhagavad Gita*, Lord Krishna tells the warrior *Arjuna*, you have a right to perform your prescribed duties, but you are not entitled to the fruits of your actions. Never consider yourself to be the cause of the results of your activities, nor be attached to inaction.[27] For most, life is a relentless march forward toward new pursuits and new goals. We think we are the creator of our will and actions, but higher forces are always at work. So too, not acting at all, or acting too soon, or without due process works against natural intelligence. In the *Tao te Ching*, Lao Tzu points out that *non-doing* doesn't mean laziness, retirement, or inertia. Inaction can brace the tranquil inner stillness that supports the moment for action.[28]

Three Techniques for Letting Go[29]

Modern psychologists can spend years with patients examining past mental habits. But rather than delve into the complex world of the mind, Vedic and Yogic approaches move the attention away from problematic subjects, removing their source of power. Rather than see our thoughts and emotions as personal, a primary function of Vedic psychology views the mental field not as ourselves, but simply as objects passing through. In doing so we can see more clearly and choose what we want to attend to, and what to let go. To discard thoughts and emotions that don't serve us, Vedic wisdom offers three main approaches: a physical and a mental method, and also meditation.

Physical techniques place the energy associated with an unwanted thought into something else. The original and best method moves the awareness from unhelpful thoughts to observe the breath—its inhale and exhale, ebb and flow. Turning the focus from unhelpful thoughts to the breath unites the body and mind, and quiets the system considerably. Other physical focuses on which to place the attention include taking a walk, *prāṇāyāma*, reading, cooking, cleaning, or another purposeful or enjoyable activity.

Mental techniques to divert the attention from redundant thoughts traditionally use the resonance of sound. The mind is redirected to repeat a *mantra* or syllable such as *ram* (good for *vāta*), *sham* or *shreem* (good for *pitta*), or *hum* (good for *kapha*). The syllable can be slowly repeated three, nine, twenty-one, one hundred and eight, or more times, or can be timed for three, five, or more minutes. The more time and focus given to a *mantra*, the more power it develops. Appropriate *mantras*, correctly pronounced, awaken intelligence, destroy *tamas*, and create *sattva*. The mind can also be redirected to a helpful affirmation or saying. Whatever your choice, focus the mind on the activity, sound,

or saying completely. A more challenging mental method rejects unwanted thoughts as they enter awareness. Like recognizing an unwelcome guest as they pass the window, we simply don't open the door. When their knock is not answered, uninvited guests go away and eventually stop coming. Even if you fail to reject a thought as it comes through the door, as soon as you notice it, use the breath, action, or sound to redirect and focus the mind's power.

We build affinities with things simply by thinking about them. When it comes to food, if we don't think about ice cream, no attraction exists. But if ice cream enters the mind, the more we dwell upon its cool, rich, moist sweetness, the more we yearn the treat. Observe the mind to recognize thoughts and actions that don't serve you and observe their triggers and consequences. Exposing unwanted thoughts and destructive habits to the light of awareness, then turning the mind away, dissolves their power and initiates the process of change. After identifying potential barriers and addressing what can be done in the external environment, turn your attention to new ways of thinking, doing, and being. At the broadest level, our actions transform when our way of being transforms—no willpower, or physical or emotional turmoil required.

Daily meditation is a third technique for letting go. Without any specific focus, with regular meditation, attachments and desires are loosened and eventually fall away. Meditation can also take the form of visualization, where we see ourselves competently performing the new habits we desire. Two, or all three techniques for letting go can be practiced concurrently.

Focusing on New and Favorable Habits

Habits of thought and action that lie low in the consciousness run on conditioned memory. But if we want something different, we need to think and act differently. Adopting fresh habits requires a shift in mental and physical momentum. Instead of mindless repetition, when the attention (and hence vital energy) are focused on what we want, and new patterns are repeated, novel nerve pathways are created, and the process of habituation begins.

Attention Alongside Repetition

From a modern scientific perspective, intense focus is a trigger that activates the *nucleus basalis*, a nub in the basal forebrain packed with essential chemicals for nerve impulse transmission. This part of the brain is most active during youth while new neural pathways are laid. During adolescence the nucleus basalis becomes less active, and in adults is thought to be dormant, unless awoken by a survival threat or similarly powerful event. But another way to activate the nucleus basalis is concentrated focus. Paying close attention to the new habits we wish to create—attention alongside repetition—makes wiring new practices easier. Mental rehearsal is useful then, focus your mind and physical being on the sensory experience of the new habit every time you perform it.

Love is also the way. In the body the essence of love penetrates deeply, to soften the matrix and make us receptive to change. One hormone highlighted in the love response is *oxytocin*. Called the *love hormone*, oxytocin is released from the brain in response to bonding experiences. In new parents, oxytocin promotes feelings of love, calm, and closeness, and helps the adoption of new patterns once parenthood has arrived. At large in society, feelings of love, connection, affection and genuine gratitude cultivate oxytocin release, and enhance positive emotions, relaxation, receptivity, and endurance.[30]

For positive change, then, the recipe is *focus* plus *love*. Attention and focus activate and power transformation, and love softens and calms our being, making it receptive to new impressions. Moving through new experiences with attention and awareness, and feelings of gratitude, freshness, and enthusiasm are powerful conduits for change.

Plus, as we practice new skills, the demand for energy decreases. And as benefits become apparent, appreciation and dedication are reinforced.

Prioritize Your Focus

Dietary and lifestyle change requires choices and decisions, but not all must be made at once. It can be enough to decide to release one old habit and introduce one new food or aspect of the meal pattern. A usefully ordered approach would first apply the medicine of negation, reducing and removing foods and eating patterns that aggravate the *dosha*. This primary step helps to uproot problems at their source. Displaced foods and routines are then replaced with balancing options.

When creating new habits, it makes sense to set S.M.A.R.T goals: specific, measurable, achievable, relevant/realistic, and time-based, such as:

- Halving the quantity of one or two problematic foods within the next month
- Buying and enjoying more whole foods and/or *sattvic* foods and/or seasonal produce every time you shop
- Try one new fresh food each week
- Cook a fresh meal from scratch at least once a week
- Practice embodied eating at one meal each day
- Eat before 7:00 p.m. at least four nights each week

It's good to be S.M.A.R.T, but flexibility is required, too. All food-based decisions are situational, dynamic, and multifaceted. Daily eating involves food acquisition, preparation, serving, chewing, tasting, digesting, and evacuating. Nutrition is an all-embracing art, not reductionist science. Short- and long-term goals can't be too rigidly structured. From an Ayurvedic perspective, all practices and routines benefit from timely adaptation. Certain choices may work in this season of the year or life, yet in a different phase or situation we are better off without them.

When eating according to *dosha* a good start may be to apply this focus to two meals in three. Or structure *dosha*-friendly breakfasts and dinners, and eat more freely (but not mindlessly) at lunch. Or eat with more structure on weekdays, and more spontaneously (but not excessively) on weekends. Focus on your goal(s), but allow needed time and space for new practices to develop. Accept that your abilities and behaviors change in different situations. Don't become attached to specific outcomes, or the way they manifest. Every day, be open to receiving different or better than what you can conceive right now. Disciplined yet responsive daily habits encourage freedom, balance, and flow.

Positive Change Takes Time

In dropping old habits, we make a positive move away from the past yet, too much change, too quickly, disturbs the entire system. For the food body, an alteration in diet means a shift in the substances that fuel, nourish, and build it. Once habituated, sudden change can cause immense harm. For this reason, don't go "cold turkey" with foods the body is adapted to and depends on. Gradual, sustainable change (i.e. one quarter of a portion each day, week, or month) is ideal. And choose your time to implement change. Stability in other areas of life can support change; equally, a phase of significant transformation, such as moving to a new job, house, or a holiday, can be a good time to insert new habits, and leave the old behind.

When it comes to behavioral habits, at a minimum it takes twenty-one days of conscious, embodied repetition for new nerve pathways and metabolic adaptations to commence. For health habits to become second nature, it may take two or three months, but can also take much longer.[31] Significant dietary change such as transitioning to a plant-based diet often takes years. Meat, and former favorite foods such as dairy, wheat, and coffee also take time for

the mind to release (yet may or may not need to be eliminated completely, and can sometimes be reintroduced in small quantities after some time). It also takes time for the tongue to enjoy foods that initially seem foreign or exotic, and for the digestive fires to adjust. Habituation to junk food—a feat probably honed since childhood—means that natural foods can lack taste and appeal. For the taste buds to recover from intense chemical onslaught and perceive the natural flavors of whole foods, it takes at least a few weeks. Bitter foods aid this process.

Today's powerful technologies and fast-paced culture have conditioned us to expect instant change; many are like spoiled children, desiring immediate gratification. But seeking greater health and wholeness is not something that slots into a few minutes each day. Healthier dietary and lifestyle choices do bring immediate feelings of well-being, but dietary change and healthy balance take weeks, months, years, and are essentially ongoing. For example, once one food is eliminated, we often become aware of other unhelpful foods. The longer new habits exist, the more likely they are to stay, and for old habits not to return. But sometimes the momentum of old habits arises. When this happens, observe them, warts and all. Rather than condemn yourself, congratulate your growing awareness. Applaud your self-honesty and commitment.

Hardened bread, milk, cheese, sugar, chocolate, junk food, soft drink, coffee, and alcohol junkies may think that reducing or removing these foods seems like an unreachable goal. But with knowledge, attention, practice, and perseverance positive change always takes place. Every day spend at least a few moments connecting with important goals. Every week put aside some time, and every few months take some hours or a whole day to review and refocus. Even though we may sometimes feel stuck, this is not the case; life is constantly unfolding. With patience and perseverance, we don't have to scale the tree to pluck the fruits of our labors; in time they ripen and fall by themselves. The benefits of positive change continue to deepen and compound over time. When the fundamentals become deeply engrained, we have a platform to build on, and grow. Transition takes effort. But with attention and practice, feelings of struggle or deprivation are replaced by increased awareness, choice, vitality, balance, and freedom.

Enjoy Social and Environmental Support

Humans are social animals. Surrounded by people, ideas, and spaces that support us, our well-being and happiness expand. In the process of health and disease, our personal relationships with other people can be highly influential. And in the process of healing and change, social and environmental support is crucial. Our relationships with parents, spouses, children, and peers can make or break long-term change. One significant enabler of change is support from family members. Call on partners and close friends. Spend time with people who can empathize or offer an ear, especially those who are mature and experienced. If change is desired, talk openly with significant others. Explain your logic and help others understand you. Greater understanding lends greater support. Spend time with like-minded people and those who are already following a similar path. Seek health practitioners, counselors, support groups, and affirming social networks that foster new ways. *Vāta* and *kapha* types particularly benefit from shared experiences. The push toward globalization has not benefitted the food supply. But global communication technologies offer new connections with countless others, rendering the world a global village. In order to enjoy the support of the environment, we need to understand it and learn to work with it. From an Ayurvedic perspective, the best way to do this is to create a custom-made daily routine.

To enjoy wider support, we also need to take care of our broader surroundings. Supporting the environment foremost includes Mother

---

Dināchārya (The Daily Routine)

The daily routine, or *dināchārya*, is one arm of *Āyurveda's* powerful triad of healthy living, alongside diet and medical therapies. A daily routine encompasses eating patterns and other actions and practices to balance the *dosha*; kindle the *agnis*; facilitate the smooth flow of *prāna*; cleanse and nourish the tissues, mind, and senses; and support wakefulness and adequate sleep. All practices should be tailored toward the individual, and adapted to the time of day, season, and local environment. A *dināchārya* is best constructed slowly over time. In general, activities within a daily routine focus on the early morning period, making use of this generative time, and setting the tone of the day. Plus, our energy and attention are generally best early on. When there are things you wish to do daily, uphold these priorities in the morning. In addition to diet, a daily routine may include one or many of the following: a set, pre-dawn time for rising; voiding the bladder and bowels; cleaning the teeth; scraping the tongue; an early morning drink; oil gargling; nasal cleansing and lubricating; eye bath or salve; oiling the ears; oil self-massage; bathing; physical exercise; yoga practices; oiling the feet; and an early, set time for sleeping. All of these practices should be tailored to one's *dosha* type and environment. Performing your chosen practices should be regular, but not be laborious. Because *like increases like*, feeling stressed, hurried, or dreamy throughout daily practices doesn't support happiness or positive change. Be attentive and nurture appreciation and a positive state of mind. Respect the practices for what they are. Dedicate them to a higher purpose. At first, creating a daily routine means there are new decisions to be made. But eventually a regular *dināchārya* entails fewer ongoing choices, accompanied by greater vitality and balance.

Earth, who does her best to support us continually and unconditionally. Tribal cultures honor this deep relationship with natural habitats, which provide all life lessons and solutions. In relation to Mother Earth we are both *child* and *custodian*. As a child we take, and as a custodian we give. Don't be purely an extractor and contribute to advanced problems of decreasing natural habitats and animal life, soil nutrient depletion and erosion, and widespread chemical pollution. In the coming century, local and global temperatures could rise anywhere from two to over ten degrees Fahrenheit.[32] Already shorelines are changing and habitable and arable lands are lost, as is biodiversity. With the assistance of *landscape amnesia* (our knack for quickly forgetting how natural landscapes originally looked), and *creeping normalcy* (slow trends concealed in noisy fluctuations),[33] coupled with heavy-handed will and greed, we find ourselves in a precarious position. As carbon dioxide levels continue to rise all living systems will be increasingly stressed and vulnerable to disease and decay. To support Mother Earth, work with local and state governments to maintain natural communal spaces such as city parks, national parks, and wilderness areas. Support forests and re-forestation. Back the creation of marine reserves in the world's seas and oceans.

The complexity of the global food chain and current food industry practices have us believe that our food choices exist as discrete entities from broader life. Yet daily food choices influence us personally and also the world at large, shaping the ways agricultural lands are used, what and how foods are grown, and where government, industry, and consumer dollars are spent. Our food choice decisions affect the lives and deaths of countless plants and animals. As the food chain has lengthened, healthy longevity has shortened, and we live in a landscape of false plenty. In recent decades, the stored sunshine captured in petroleum has been pumped into every level of food production. Yet, with less or no petroleum, the global food system falls apart. Other problems include depleted soils, the disappearance of pollinators (especially bees and butterflies), expanding human populations that inhabit viable croplands yet also need more food, and increasing affluence leading to greater demand for foods and comforts, in the face of deceasing

supplies. Plus, the failing health of many individuals, societies, and the planetary ecosystem as a whole. For now, enough food may be available, affordable, and convenient, but future food security and access to genuinely good food and water are foreseeable challenges. Moving a majority of food procurement back to local, sustainable food systems is a global imperative.

To support the social and ecological environments you live in, start in your own backyard by planting fruit trees or growing veggies or herbs in pots. Buy foods grown using regenerative agriculture that creates topsoil and improves land, rather than methods that destroy and waste soils and life. Reduce. Reuse. Recycle. Support food chains that recognize and adhere to natural laws, respect plants and animals, and allow farmers to have their say. Support businesses that make fresh, local, and organic food available, and the policies that back them. Look at new technologies and the ways they are (and are not) regulated. Expect a higher standard of the food we have available. Contact food companies and food regulating bodies to make them accountable and have your say. Today's meal choices influence the foods available to fill our plates tomorrow. Food producers, manufacturers, and retailers respond to customer demand. Vote with your fork, finances, and feet.

Conclusion

To understand ourselves and be healthy, Western science teaches us to look outside to specialized people and technologies, to divide organs from integrated systems, nutrients from food complexes, the mental from the physical, rational thought from personal feelings. To try to understand life we have been taught to pull things apart—then we forget to reassemble them again, or simply don't know how. Division promotes temporary clarity, but destroys collective existence.

Āyurveda encourages each individual to find their own path, and fully connect with and contribute to life. The Sanskrit word for health, *svastha*, means to be wholly situated within oneself; to know oneself. And the English words *whole, health,* and *healing* derive from the same etymological root. True health is a state of wholeness within ourselves, a natural and connected state. We are not a solid, stable structure, but a dynamic assemblage of energy and intelligence within the energy and intelligence of larger cosmic field. People, objects, and elements are different, but they are not separate. As healthy individuals we become a complete entity, existing in a unified field.

Overall, the *Charaka Samhitā* considers health to exist when:

- The three *doshas* are in equilibrium
- All body tissues function as intended
- The appetite is regular and the digestive fires are balanced
- Wastes are properly formed and completely eliminated
- All physical and subtle channels flow unhindered, including the subtle life-force *prāna*
- The five senses function well
- The mind has clarity and can discern

- Physical and subtle processes are integrated
- Happiness is a dominant emotion
- The individual is established in their spiritual nature

For each of us, the path toward dynamic balance is different depending on our unique constitution, and individual history, tendencies, and life situation. Our passage is also influenced by our level of access to supportive information and resources, our level of knowledge and skill acquisition, and available time, confidence, and commitment. In health and life, it may not be possible to attain harmony at all levels, but to realize greater balance we can work toward any health goal. All efforts in the direction of balance affect every aspect and contribute to greater intrinsic intelligence. The food body needs nourishment and balanced expression, but so does the mind and its senses, the heart, and the energy system, wisdom body, and spirit. The *Charaka Samhitā* emphasizes that health and longevity is supported when there is a balance between vibrant physical, mental, and spiritual being. *Āyurveda* dedicates most efforts toward balancing and enlivening the physical body. But its ultimate purpose is to fortify and integrate the physical body in order to move beyond it and experience more subtle realms.

In order to elevate every level of being, the science and art of Ayurvedic nutrition emphasizes savoring fresh, local, whole foods that are readily digestible and include all six tastes in proportions that balance one's constitution, within organized, responsive living. Health is supported when we avoid foods high in the qualities we already possess and choose nourishing foods that provide more of the qualities we lack. We move toward ongoing health, balance, and freedom by observing and living in accordance with natural cycles and changing inner and outer events; supporting the intelligence of the *dosha* and physical body; nurturing the quality of *sattva*; being disciplined yet responsive and flexible; and fostering experience and feeling. Ayurvedic traditions also understand that the food we eat intimately mingles with the mind, and that reverent and wholesome eating is an instrument and expression of integral living. By complementing the body's natural metabolism, food becomes therapy. Chosen intelligently (rather than out of habit or compulsion), balanced eating patterns cure or improve most physical disease conditions, and elevate every level of life.

Āyurveda treats individuals. Plus, the more attention we pay, the better equipped we become to treat ourselves. Rather than a medical system, the time-tested self-healing wisdom of *Āyurveda* is intended for those willing to take responsibility for themselves and their perpetual relationships. The guiding principles and practices of *Āyurveda* offer self-understanding deeper than the everyday level. Working with the three *dosha* and our unique constitution, we are offered a methodology for self-awareness, self-healing, and creation of well-rounded health—the highest level of which is to eradicate the cause(s) of imbalance before disease manifests. Overall the healing approach of *Āyurveda* places emphasis on supportive diet, daily routine, and medical and herbal therapies. When these approaches are combined, health benefits accumulate—one plus one plus one equals eight. If, however, you're not sure what to do, then do nothing, or stop doing things that aggravate imbalance. Over time, through self-observation, practice, experimentation, and personal experience, understanding grows. At every stage, further reading and the guidance of an Ayurvedic practitioner can offer even more valuable insights.

Humans have been given free will to decide the direction of their senses and life energies, but too often we squander this liberty on mindless habits and blind beliefs. Handing responsibility to mechanical routines, computer-generated intelligence, squanders our uniqueness and gives away our free will. Desire to change and true freedom to change may seem poles apart, but ultimately both are states of mind. We can be bound up in past patterns, or we can cultivate freedom by questioning our beliefs and conditionings, and letting go what no longer serves us. Meaningless ideas and routines are anti-life and anti-transformation, but through the lens of *Āyurveda*, each decision becomes an opportunity for positive growth.

By consciously moving into greater alignment, we line up with the flow of existence, personal powers and truths are amplified, and life is an instrument of joy and freedom. When the system is balanced, the food body knows that *opposites reduce*. Out of balance, we fall prey to the universal law *like attracts like*. But we can also use this law to our advantage. According to this principle, the world is like an echo—whatever we put out there returns. In life and in health, we eternally reap what we sow.

Appendix J: Cooking Tips

Preparing Pulses and Whole Grains

Well-prepared beans, lentils, and whole grains make a tasty, nutritious addition to the diet of all constitutions. For excellent digestion and satisfaction:

- *Pre-soak overnight one-part beans/whole grains in four parts water.* Soak large beans at least twelve hours; whole grains eight hours; lentils two to four hours. Pre-soaking wakes seeds up, softens and swells, and stimulates enzymes that break down toxins and nutrient complexes. To enhance this process, add a fermenting medium to the soak water, such as a few teaspoons of whey (the clear liquid in yogurt), or apple cider vinegar. Rinse before cooking.
- *Cook thoroughly.* In a pot, simmer kidney and lima beans for more than two hours. Parboiling and changing the water once or twice helps to reduce their gas-forming properties. In a pressure cooker, toot ten to twelve times (Indian pressure cookers "toot") or jingle for fifteen minutes (Western pressure cooker's usually "jingle"). For lentils and whole grains, simmer in a pot for thirty to forty-five minutes. In a large pressure cooker, toot two or three times, or jingle for five minutes.
- *Add herbs and spices, and other digestive and softening agents to cooking,* such as a half to one teaspoon of turmeric, fennel, and/or cumin seeds; garlic; onions; ginger root; bay leaves; and a pinch of asafoetida (*hing*), or baking soda.
- *Eat small amounts and chew thoroughly.* Start slowly if approaching legumes or whole grains for the first time. Begin with a few tablespoons within a warm salad or meal.

- Choose legumes that suit your constitution and digestive capacity.
- *Eat freshly cooked.* If you have leftovers, reheat well and add extra moisture (water; *ghee*) and ginger root to add digestive fire. Leftovers are harder to digest.
- *Sprout seeds.* Soak seeds such as green mung beans or alfalfa in a covered, darkened jar for twelve hours. Fasten a thin cloth or gauze over the mouth, and drain. Expose to daylight. Rinse and drain a few times a day for two to three days. Sprinkle sprouts over cooked meals, or lightly steamed in mixed dishes.

Kitchari

Kitchari is easy to cook, readily digestible, nourishing, balancing, and cleansing for all *dosha* types. Here is a basic everyday recipe, plus ideas to substitute and mix different pulses and grains, vegetables, and spices.

Serves: 4

Ingredients for the pot:
   1½ cups split mung beans
   1 cup basmati rice
   2 tsp *ghee* or oil

   ½ tsp turmeric
   ½ tsp unrefined salt
   1 pinch asafoetida (*hing*)
   6 cups water (add extra ½ cup if grains not pre-soaked)

Ingredients for tadka—a technique of tempering spices to add extra flavor and digestibility:
   2 tsp *ghee*
   2 tsp sesame oil
   1 tsp whole or ground seeds of cumin
   ½ tsp fennel seeds
   ½ tsp mustard seeds
   ½ tsp ajowan seeds
   ½ tsp fenugreek seeds

Basic preparation:
1. Rinse and drain grains and place in a pressure cooker or cookpot with all other pot ingredients (not the *tadka* ingredients). Fit lid and place over medium heat.
2. If using a pressure cooker, allow the vessel to come to pressure for a few toots, or jingle for five minutes (a little longer if the grains are not pre-soaked). Remove from heat and allow to stand for ten minutes. If pot cooking, cover and bring to boil then reduce to a simmer for twenty minutes. Add more water if necessary.

3. While the grains cook, make the *tadka*[13] in a heavy-bottomed pan. Warm the *ghee* and oil over low heat. Add the seeds and lightly toast until the mustard kernels pop, the fenugreek seed turn dark brown (not black or they become bitter!), and the pan is aromatic. Add any powdered spices. Add a pinch of salt here also, if you are adding onions or tomatoes (see later variations). Stir and allow to gently sizzle for a few minutes, then cover and remove from heat.

4. When the grains are ready, keep them simmering, and stir in the *tadka*. Adjust seasoning to taste.

5. Replace the lid, remove the *kitchari* from the flame, and allow it to stand five minutes before serving.

Variations:

During modified fasting or convalescence use rice and mung dal in a ratio of 2:1 or 3:1. Reduce seasoning to turmeric, cumin seeds, and salt.

In daily meals, use different varieties of lentils—red, yellow, brown, and rice—long grain, short grain, brown, red. Mix different combinations of lentils or rice together.

Add chopped vegetables such as carrots, green beans, peas, cauliflower, or squash while cooking the grains. For pot cooking add vegetables at any stage—hard vegetables earlier, and soft veggies toward the end.

Add additional spices to the *tadka* such as chili, black pepper, bay leaves, ginger root, or garlic. And ingredients (after the spices are roasted) such as diced or sliced onion, tomato, mushrooms, zucchini, spinach, or kale. In general, add only one or two different vegetables; too many confuses the flavors.

Serve with a generous squeeze of lemon or lime or dollop of fresh herb chutney. *Vāta* types can add extra *ghee*; oil; salt. *Pitta* types can add *ghee*; sliced cucumber; fresh coriander; salad greens. *Kapha* types might like fresh chili or ginger root; black pepper; fresh herbs; salad greens.

To make a lentil curry, or dal, simply exclude the rice and reduce the water to 4½ cups. Use one, two, or a mix of lentil varieties. You can reduce the spice quantities, or leave as stated.

Simple Savory Pancakes

These thin savory pancakes are dense, nourishing, cleansing, tasty, and suitable for all *dosha* types. They are a wheat-free substitute for flat and yeasted breads. Ideal for a quick meal, accompanied by cooked vegetables, salad, soup, an omelet, or fresh chutney.

---

13 The *tadka* can also be fried first then cooked in with the grains. For convenience, fry the *tadka* in the same vessel you will cook the grains.

Makes: 5 medium-sized pancakes

Ingredients:

½ cup basmati rice

½ cup green mung dal (this is yellow split mung with the skin still on)

2 tsp chopped ginger

½ tsp turmeric

½ tsp mineral salt

A pinch of asafoetida (*hing*)

½ cup water (approx.)

A little *ghee* or oil while cooking

Basic preparation:

1. Soak the rice and mung dal in plenty of water. Cover and place on a counter for four hours. Or you can place them in the fridge and soak for eight hours or so over the day (or night).
2. Drain, rinse, and place the grains in a grinder along with all ingredients. Add water as required to make a medium-thick batter.
3. Heat a flat nonstick pan over a medium heat. When hot, if desired, spread a thin coating of *ghee* or sesame oil on the bottom.
4. Pour or scoop between ¼ to ½ cup of batter onto the pan. Use the rounded bottom of ladle or spoon to spread the batter from the center outward in a spiral pattern to make a thin round pancake.

5. When the top is dry and the bottom is dark golden brown, the pancake is ready.
6. Fold in half and serve hot.
7. Store any unused batter in the fridge in a sealed container for up to twenty-four hours.

Variations:

Try other types of rice, or a mix of rice grains. Whole grain rice needs additional soaking.

While cooking, add some grated carrot, chopped onion, tomato, or fresh herbs on top.

South Indian Coconut Vegetable Curry (*A "Thoran" from Kerala*)

This simple, versatile, tasty dish often uses just a single vegetable. Choose beetroot, cabbage, carrot, cauliflower, pumpkin, summer squash, green beans, drumsticks (moringa seed pods), spinach, or okra, or try a mix. For a simple meal, pair it with rice or another whole grain, savory pancakes, and/or lentil curry. Or include as a side-dish. It can be modified to suit all *dosha* types.

Serves: 2 as a primary constituent, or 4 as a side-dish

Ingredients:

Vegetables:

3 cups of diced vegetable

¼ tsp turmeric

¼ tsp mineral salt

Coconut mixture:

½ cup ground or shredded coconut, fresh or dried

2 tsp fresh ginger, chopped

1 fresh green chili, chopped

½ tsp cumin (whole seeds to grind, or powder)

***Tadka* (tempering the spices):**

1 tsp coconut oil

½ tsp mustard seeds

8–10 curry leaves

1 medium onion, finely diced

Mineral salt, to taste

Fresh cilantro to garnish (optional)

Basic preparation:

1. Square dice or finely chop vegetables.
2. Sprinkle over the turmeric and mineral salt to lightly coat.
3. Steam vegetables in a little water for ten to twenty minutes, until cooked.
4. While vegetables are cooking, grind or blend the coconut mixture—shredded coconut, sliced ginger, green chili, and cumin to a rough paste. If using dried coconut, allow the mixture to sit five minutes, then pulse again. Add a little water, if required.
5. To temper the spices—heat the oil in a pan over a moderate flame. When hot, add the mustard seeds and curry leaves, and gently stir until the mustard seeds pop.

6. Add the finely diced onion and stir for a few minutes to soften and give color. Then cover and remove the *tadka* from heat.
7. When the vegetables are cooked, stir the coconut mixture through, and bring to a simmer. Remove from heat.
8. Mix through the tempered spices.
9. Salt to taste.
10. Sprinkle with fresh, chopped cilantro, and serve immediately.

Variations:

Kapha types or those wanting more pungency can mix a second chopped chili, or 1 tsp of black pepper, or a clove or two of garlic in with the coconut mix.

Pitta types can omit the chili. And stir through additional fresh cilantro.

Vāta types might like to add 1 cup of natural yogurt or 1 tsp of tamarind paste when adding the coconut mixture to the cooked vegetables.

Fresh Cilantro Chutney

Chutneys made from fresh green herbs are mostly cooling, refreshing, and digestive. Plus, they pack a big nutrition and taste punch into a small serving. This fresh cilantro chutney is especially soothing for *pitta*, and balances all *doshas* in the summer heat. It adds zest and flavor to grain, vegetable, and meat dishes, and perfectly complements savory pancakes.

Serves 4

Ingredients:
   1 cup chopped cilantro leaves and soft stems
   (firmly-packed)
   2 tsp chopped ginger
   1 tsp fresh lime or lemon juice
   ½ medium orange, de-seeded (or ¼ cup thick
   orange juice)
   3 large dates, de-seeded, chopped
   ½ tsp cumin powder
   ¼ tsp mineral salt

Basic preparation:
1. Wash the cilantro.
2. Combine all ingredients in a blender and
    mix to a smooth paste. Adjust seasoning
    (salt, unrefined sugar), if required.
3. Serve immediately.
4. Store leftovers in the fridge in a non-
    reactive, sealed container for up to two days.

Variations:
Use a combination of 2 parts cilantro and 1 part
mint.

Kapha types and those wanting warmth and
spice can add a green chili, or black pepper.

Plain, Sweet, Salt, and Spiced *Lassi*[14]

Yogurt is sour, sweet, and astringent in taste,
with a hot potency, and a sour, building post-digestive effect. In general, yogurt is heavy and
congesting, but churning yogurt with water
breaks down its dense, thick structure to make
it lighter, more digestible, less mucus forming,
and beneficial for all *dosha* types. By adding
other ingredients its nature can be further aug-
mented (but be mindful of incompatible food
combinations, such as bananas and mango). In
general, *lassi* is considered digestive, nutritious,
therapeutic, and the best among milk products—
but don't drink it every day, or at night, or in winter or spring, as it is likely to become congestive.
Consume at room temperature, ideally before or
after lunch.

Ingredients:
   Freshly cultured, natural yogurt
   Room temperature water
   Sweeteners, salt, and spices as appropriate,
   suggested below

Basic preparation and variations:
1. A basic *lassi* preparation entails blending
    equal parts of yogurt and water. This may
    best suit *vāta* types, but is heavier to digest.

---

14   *Lassi* can also be called buttermilk. But traditional buttermilk is the clear liquid that remains after thick curd
is churned to butter.

For a weak *vāta* digestion, and for *pitta* and *kapha* types, use a ratio of 1:2 or 1:3 or 1:4 parts yogurt to water.

2. Blend for one to two minutes.
3. Skim off the fatty foam on top and mix in a pinch of ginger powder and cumin powder, according to taste.

To modify, or in general, *vāta* types can also add a pinch of unrefined sugar or salt.

Pitta types can add jaggery, unrefined sugar, or maple syrup; or fresh cilantro or mint; or mild powdered spices such as cardamom or coriander. They can substitute ginger powder for fresh ginger or ginger juice.

Kapha types should dilute well, and add pungent spices such as extra dry ginger, or black pepper. If sweetness is required, add a little honey.

Versions of classic recipes include:

Pachak (digestive) *Lassi*

¼ cup yogurt
¾ cup water
⅛–¼ tsp ginger powder
½ tsp cumin seeds or powder
A good pinch of rock salt
2 tsp chopped coriander to garnish

Supports the digestive fires and helps to balance all *doshas*. Take after lunch.

Sweet *Lassi*

¼ cup yogurt
¾ cup water
¼ tsp cardamom powder
1–2 tbsp unrefined sugar (to taste)
1 drop of rosewater or blend in 5 or 6 rose petals

Cooling for *pitta dosha* and refreshing for all *dosha* types in the summer heat.

Acknowledgments

I am indebted to countless teachers who have generously shared their wisdom, especially the expertise of Vaidya Atreya Smith and Dr. Sunil Joshi, and the holy sages and past Ayurvedic scholars and physicians who received and kept the illuminated teachings alive. I am also enormously grateful for: the friendship and inspiration of Michele "Atma" Gregory, Annet Hoek, and Melanie Voevodin for her wonderful suggestions, rants, and musings; to Nicole Mele, my editor at Skyhorse Publishing, for her clarity of vision, and for giving the book wings; to my sister, Lisa Colles, for helping me find my voice; to my parents, Lois and Brian, for their unconditional lifelong support; and to my husband, Digonta, for his true, unbounded love. And to Ma—Mother Nature and Mother Earth—for all creation and all healing.

Bibliography

Acharya Shunya. *Ayurveda Lifestyle Wisdom.* Colorado, Sounds True; 2017.

Caldecott, T. *Ayurveda: The Divine Science of Life.* Mosby Elsevier, 2006.

Dash, B. and Sharma, R. K. (transl.) *Caraka Saṁhitā,* vols; I—VII, Varanasi, Chowkhamba Sanskrit Series; 2015 reprint.

Dash, B. *Materia Medica of Ayurveda;* Based on Madanapala's Nighantu. New Delhi, Health harmony; 2006 reprint.

Frawley, D. *Ayurveda and the Mind: The healing of Consciousness.* New Delhi, Motilal Banarsidass; 1998.

Joshi, S. *Ayurveda and Panchakarma: The Science of Healing and Rejuvenation.* New Delhi, Motilal Banarsidass; 1998.

Lad, V. *Ayurveda. The Science of Self-Healing.* Santa Fe, NM, Lotus Press; 1984. *

Lad, U. and V. *Ayurvedic Cooking for Self-Healing.* New Delhi, Motilal Banarsidass; 1994. *

Maharaj, Nisargadatta. *I Am That.* Mumbai, Sundaram; 1973.

Morningstar, A. with Desai, U. *The Ayurvedic Cookbook.* New Delhi, Motilal Banarsidass; 1990. *

Murthy, S. K. (transl.) *Astanga Hrdayam,* vols–I—III, Varanasi, Krishnadas Academy; 1996.

Murthy, S. K. (transl.) *Bhāvaprakāśā,* vols–II, Varanasi, Krishnadas Academy; 1998.

Osho. *The Book of Secrets.* New York, St Martin's Press; 2010.

Pritchard, P. *Healing with Whole Foods: Asian Traditions and Modern Nutrition.* 3rd Edition. Berkeley CA; 2002.

Sadhguru. *Inner Engineering. A Yogi's Guide to Joy.* Penguin Ananda; 2016.

Smith, A. *The Psychology of Transformation in Yoga.* Create Space; 2013.

Smith, A. *Ayurvedic Medicine for Westerners,* vols 1–5, Switzerland, EIVS GmbH; 2000-2015.

Smith, A. *Ayurvedic Practitioners E-Learning and Practical Program Part 1, 2 & 3*. Certification Course. European Institute of Vedic Studies; 2014–2016.

Sogyal Rinpoche. *The Tibetan Book of Living and Dying*. HarperOne; 2009.

Svoboda, R. *Life, Health and Longevity*. India, Penguin; 1992.

Svoboda, R. *Prakriti: Your Ayurvedic Constitution*. New Delhi, Motilal Banarsidass; 1989.

Tirtha, Swami Sada Shiva. *The Ayurveda Encyclopedia: Natural Secrets to Healing, Prevention & Longevity*. New Delhi, Health Harmony; 1996.

Tiwari, M. Ayurveda: *A Life of Balance*. Vermont, Healing Arts Press; 1994.

Tzu, Lao. *The Tao Te Ching*. Translation by Ralph Alan Dale. London, Sacred Texts; 2002.

Welch, C. and Stillman, C. *Healthier Hormones*. E-Course. 2018.

These books offer lists indicating the thermal potency of foods.

References

1 Taittirīya *Upanishad*, 3.2.

2 See the work of Walter Jehne, climate scientist and soil microbiologist, founder and director of Healthy Soils Australia. For example: https://vimeo.com/251739209.

3 See the *Samkhya Darshana*, one of the six systems of Indian philosophy, that explains the evolution of experience from subtle form into solid matter.

4 Montgomery, D. "Growing a Revolution: Bringing Our Soil Back to Life". (2017); W. W. Norton.

5 Freed, D. "Do dietary lectins cause disease?" *BMJ*. 318; 1023-4, 1999; https://www.ncbi.nlm.nih.gov/pmc/articles/PMC1115436/pdf/1023.pdf.

6 See Nestle, M. "Food Politics: How the Food Industry Influences Nutrition and Health". (2003); University of California Press.

7 Rona R. *et al.* "The prevalence of food allergy: a meta-analysis." *J Allergy Clin Immunol.* 2007; 120:638-46. doi:10.1016/j.jaci.2007.05.026.

8 Lanou, A. Should dairy be recommended as part of a healthy vegetarian diet? Counterpoint. *Am J Clin Nutr.* 2009; 89(5):1638S-1642S. doi:10.3945/ajcn.2009.26736P.

9 Agranoff, B. and Goldberg, D. "Diet and the geographical distribution of multiple sclerosis" *Lancet.* 1974; 2(7888) doi:https://doi.org/10.1016/S0140-6736(74)92163-1.

10 Gerstein HC. "Cow's milk exposure and Type 1 diabetes mellitus: a critical review of the clinical literature." *Diabetes Care.* 1994; 17:13-19. https://doi.org/10.2337/diacare.17.1.13.

11 Sekirov I. *et al.* "Gut Microbiota in Health and Disease." *Physiol Rev.* 90; 859 –904, 2010; doi:10.1152/physrev.00045.2009.

12 Crinnion, W. and Pizzorno, J. Clinical Environmental Medicine: Identification and Natural Treatment of Diseases Caused by Common Pollutants. (2018); Elsevier.

13 https://www.who.int/news-room/fact-sheets/detail/obesity-and-overweight.

14 Osho, "The Tantra Experience: Evolution through Love". (2012); Osho Media International.

15 Woods, S. and D'Alessio, D. "Central Control of Body Weight and Appetite". *J Clinical Endo Metab*, 2008; Volume 93(11): s37-s50. https://doi.org/10.1210/jc.2008-1630.

16 See Katz, S. E. "The Art of Fermentation: An In-Depth Exploration of Essential Concepts and Processes from Around the World". (2012); Chelsea Green Publishing.

17 Surapala; Verses 1.1-4; 8.

18 McGonigal, K. (Sep, 2013). How to make stress your friend [Video file]. Viewed 22 Jan 2020. Retrieved from https://www.ted.com/speakers/kelly_mcgonigal.

19 Wansink, B. *et al.* "Internal and External Cues of Meal Cessation: The French Paradox Redux?". *Obesity*. 2007; Volume 15(12):2920-2924. https://doi.org/10.1038/oby.2007.348.

20 Alonso-Alonso, M *et al.* "Food reward system: current perspectives and future research needs" *Nutrition Reviews*, 2015; 73(5):296-307. https://doi.org/10.1093/nutrit/nuv002.

21 Chandra Bose, J. "The Nervous Mechanism of Plants". (1926); Longmans Green.

22 Backster, C. "Primary Perception: Bio-communication with Plants, Living Foods, and Human Cells". (2003); White Rose Millennium Pr. Findly, E.

23 Ibid.

24 Jung, C. G. "Personality Types". (1921); Princeton University Press (1976).

25 Taittirīya *Upanishad*, 3.2.

26 Bandura, A. "Social foundations of thought and action: a social cognitive theory". (1986); Englewood Cliffs, N.J.: Prentice-Hall.

27 Verse 2.47.

28 Lao Tzu. "The Tao te Ching", Translation by Ralph Alan Dale. (2002); London, Duncan Baird Publishers. Verses 16 and 48.

29 These techniques were taught to me by my teacher, Vaidya Atreya Smith, who learned them from his teacher, Sri H.W.L Poonjaji.

30 Magon, N. and Kalra, S. "The orgasmic history of oxytocin: Love, lust, and labor" *Indian J Endocrinol Metab*; 2011; 15(Suppl3): S156-S161. doi:10.4103/2230-8210.84851.

31 Lally, P. *et al.* "How are habits formed: Modelling habit formation in the real world" *Eur J Soc Psych*. 2010; 40(6):998-1009. https://doi.org/10.1002/ejsp.674.

32 Global Climate Change: Effects. NASA Global Climate Change: Vital Signs of the Planet. June 15, 2008. Viewed 22 Jan 2020. Retrieved from https://climate.nasa.gov/effects/.

33 Diamond, J. "Collapse: How Societies Choose to Fail or Succeed". (2005); Penguin Books Ltd.

Index